Adolescent Nutrition

CURRENT CONCEPTS IN NUTRITION

Myron Winick, Editor

Institute of Human Nutrition
Columbia University College of Physicians and Surgeons

ADOLESCENT NUTRITION

Edited by

MYRON WINICK
Institute of Human Nutrition
Columbia University College of Physicians and Surgeons

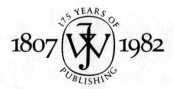

175 YEARS OF PUBLISHING
1807 1982

A Wiley-Interscience Publication

JOHN WILEY & SONS
New York • Chichester • Brisbane • Toronto • Singapore

Copyright © 1982 by John Wiley & Sons, Inc.

All rights reserved. Published simultaneously in Canada.

Reproduction or translation of any part of this work
beyond that permitted by Section 107 or 108 of the
1976 United States Copyright Act without the permission
of the copyright owner is unlawful. Requests for
permission or further information should be addressed to
the Permissions Department, John Wiley & Sons, Inc.

Library of Congress Cataloging in Publication Data:

Main entry under title:

Adolescent nutrition.

  (Current concepts in nutrition, ISSN 0090-0443; v. 11)
  "A Wiley-Interscience publication."
  Includes index.
  1. Youth—Nutrition.   I. Winick, Myron.
II. Series.
TX361.Y6A36   613.2'088055   81-19748
ISBN 0-471-86543-5   AACR2

Printed in the United States of America

10 9 8 7 6 5 4 3 2 1

Preface

Adolescence is a period of marked change, a period during which the individual rapidly undergoes a series of sequential physical and mental changes that transform a small child into a young adult. This volume has been oganized to document these changes, explore the mechanisms by which they occur, and examine the effects of altered nutritional states on the sequence of adolescence and its ultimate outcome.

Part 1 examines the normal adolescent. Chapter 1 describes the endocrine changes that occur in both boys and girls which initiate the entrance into adolescence and which govern the changes that occur. Chapter 2 focuses on the changes in body composition accompanying adolescence in both boys and girls. These changes are very different in the two sexes, boys depositing mostly muscle whereas girls deposit mostly fat, and therefore the nutritional requirements will differ in boys and girls. These requirements are considered in Chapter 3. The concept of sex maturity index is introduced—a method of assessing the stage of adolescence, independent of age, in both boys and girls. Although the sequence of events in both sexes follows a relatively fixed schedule once initiated, the time of initiation of adolescence may vary widely. Thus the *average* girl begins her growth spurt around age twelve but this can vary from as early as nine to as late as sixteen. In boys the average age is two years later but again the spread may be very wide. In considering nutritional requirements it is the stage rather than the chronological age that is important. For example, iron deficiency is most likely to occur after the growth spurt begins in boys and can be exaggerated after menstruation begins in girls.

The adolescent in our society is subjected to various stresses. Part 2 discusses two of the most common: pregnancy and lactation, and competitive sports. In both of these situations requirements for all nutrients increase. The increase, however, is specific for the stress that is being imposed, for it must take care of the particular condition while at the same time allowing the adolescent to grow.

Part 3 describes the two most prevalent specific deficiencies encountered by adolescents: iron deficiency and zinc deficiency. Both of these deficiencies occur because of the increased demands imposed by rapid growth and both can cause troublesome and sometimes extremely serious symptoms.

Part 4 discusses the nutritional management of certain diseases that are common in adolescents. The discussion of Keshan Disease by Dr. Keyou Ge of the Institute of Health of the Chinese Academy of Medicine is a classic description of the discovery of a specific nutrient deficiency in a large population which was resulting in widespread mortality and morbidity and the public health measures taken to eradicate the disease. The chapter on anorexia nervosa covers both the nutritional and psychiatric management of this disease. The importance of team management is emphasized. The same is true in the obese adolescent.

Chronic bowel disease can be effectively treated medically by dietary means but care must be taken to avoid undernutrition and subsequent growth failure. Steroids should be used with great caution because of their potential growth stunting effects. Finally, some new data are presented which suggest that saturated fat may not be the only dietary component to increase the risk for coronary artery disease.

Taken in its entirety, this volume covers the nutritional needs of adolescents under a variety of circumstances during health and disease. I hope the new information it includes will lead to new discoveries for the scientist and fresh treatment approaches for the practitioner.

MYRON WINICK

New York, New York
January 1982

Contents

PART 4   NUTRITION IN DISEASES COMMON IN ADOLESCENCE

Adolescent Nutrition

PART 1

Normal Nutrition

1

Nutrition and the Neuroendocrinology of Puberty

JEREMY S. D. WINTER

University of Manitoba, and Children's Hospital of Winnipeg, Winnipeg, Manitoba, Canada

Puberty is one phase in a process of neuroendocrine maturation which begins in early fetal life and continues through to adulthood (Figure 1-1). Not surprisingly this process can be influenced by external factors, one of the most important of which is the level of nutrition.

One sign of this influence has been the secular trend in Western industrialized nations to earlier puberty as well as to more rapid physical growth. Between 1850 and 1950 the mean age of menarche decreased by 3 to 4 months each decade, a trend that has only levelled off in the last 20 years. In North America today most girls begin breast and sex hair development between 8 and 13 years of age, and experience menarche about 2½ years later (with considerable individual variation). In boys, testicular enlargement begins between 9 and 14 years of age, and other secondary sexual characteristics appear over the next 2 to 2½ years.

THE DEVELOPMENT OF THE REPRODUCTIVE ENDOCRINE SYSTEM

The Fetus

The first sign of sexually dimorphic development is the appearance in the 6-week male fetus of testes. Under the initial stimulus of chorionic

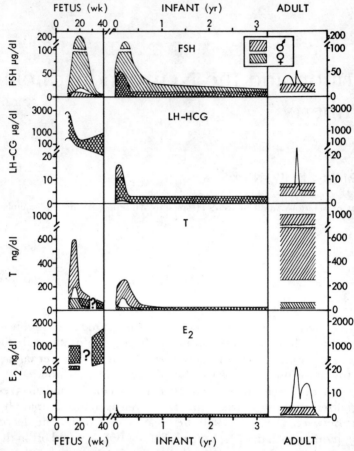

Figure 1-1.   A schematic summary of the changes in serum concentrations of FSH, LH (plus HCG during fetal life), testosterone (T), and estradiol (E₂) from conception to adult life in males and females. Serum FSH and LH concentrations are in μg LER-907/dl. The adult segment compares the male range with female values during one typical menstrual cycle.

gonadotropin these secrete testosterone in amounts sufficient to raise serum levels to the adult male range and to induce masculine differentiation of the internal and external genitalia (1). The fetal ovaries develop somewhat later and do not play a similar essential role in female genital differentiation; however, by midpregnancy the fetal ovary contains large numbers of follicles and is producing some sex steroids.

As the gonads develop, so too do those structures which will ultimately regulate their function. The fetal pituitary begins to secrete FSH and LH by 10 weeks gestation. Serum concentrations of these hormones rise to a peak at 16 to 18 weeks and then decline; levels in midpregnancy are considerably higher in females than in males. At the same time one can identify in the hypothalamus neurons containing gonadotropin-releasing hormone (GnRH), the axons of which terminate in the median eminence. Hypothalamic levels of GnRH increase during the first half of pregnancy in parallel to the rise in gonadotropin secretion, but no sex difference such as that seen with FSH and LH is observed (2). Recent studies in our laboratory have demonstrated that functional capillary connections exist between the median eminence and the anterior pituitary as early as 11 weeks gestation, while other studies have shown that the fetal pituitary is responsive to GnRH stimulation. These observations suggest that fetal pituitary gonadotropin secretion is under hypothalamic regulation from its inception. In turn, fetal pituitary gonadotropins appear to be essential for normal gonadal endocrine function and germ cell maturation.

After midpregnancy there is a decline in serum FSH and LH concentrations which likely reflects maturation of a negative feedback system responsive to the high levels of placental estrogens, and/or progesterone. The lower values of serum gonadotropins in male fetuses during the second trimester suggest that even at this early stage fetal pituitary function is modulated in part by testicular androgens.

The Infant

By the time of birth the reproductive endocrine system is structurally complete, although the mechanisms that regulate GnRH and gonadotropin secretion will continue to mature through childhood and adolescence. The disappearance from the neonatal circulation of placental estrogens removes their negative feedback influence and triggers in all infants a brisk increase in gonadotropin secretion (3). In males the testis responds with a parallel rise in testosterone secretion, which in turn somewhat blunts the gonadotropin rise (Figure 1-1). However in infant girls the ovarian steroidogenic response is less prominent; female serum gonadotropin levels often reach the postmenopausal range during the first year of life and may not return to the usual prepubertal range until 3 or 4 years of age.

Childhood

The decade between infancy and puberty is characterized by low levels of gonadotropin and sex steroid secretion. However, both the pituitary and the gonads of the child are capable of adult endocrine function; their relative dormancy results from the interaction of two mechanisms that serve to inhibit the pulsatile secretion of hypothalamic GnRH (Figure 1-2). The first of these is a poorly understood CNS inhibitory mechanism which may be analogous to that which mediates reproductive inactivity through a kind of reverse puberty in seasonal breeding species, such as the sheep. This neuroendocrine system serves as an intrinsic biological clock, but its function can be modulated by external influences such as nutrition, the light–dark cycle, and sex steroids.

The second mechanism involves feedback inhibition by sex steroids, to the action of which the prepubertal hypothalamus is remarkably sensitive. The interaction of these two mechanisms can be seen in agonadal children, who show high levels of serum gonadotropins in infancy, a decline during childhood, and then a final rise to adult castrate levels at about age 12 (4).

During late childhood there is a gradual increase in adrenal secretion of C-19 steroids such as dehydroepiandrosterone and androstenedione. This phenomenon, termed adrenarche, may reflect either changes in pituitary function or merely intrinsic changes in adrenal steroidogenesis as a function of growth (5). Some authors, having observed that excessive amounts of potent androgen can accelerate hypothalamic maturation and thus the onset of puberty, have postulated a similar physiological role for these weak adrenal androgens, but there is little clinical or experimental support for such a relationship.

Puberty

The onset of puberty is signalled by a reduction in central inhibition of pulsatile hypothalamic GnRH secretion, which is first reflected in episodic sleep-associated bursts of gonadotropin release (6). The endocrine system amplifies this initial neural signal with time, so the pituitary becomes increasingly responsive to GnRH, and the gonads more sensitive to gonadotropic stimulation. At the same time, but probably as a secondary phenomenon, the hypothalamus and pituitary become less sensitive to feedback inhibition by gonadal steroids.

As puberty progresses sleep-associated pituitary activity is replaced by the adult pattern of pulsatile gonadotropin secretion approximately every 2 hours throughout the day and night. Mean serum concentrations of FSH and LH rise (7) and in turn elicit rising levels of gonadal androgens and estrogens (Figures 1-3 and 1-4). These sex steroids not only cause the appearance of secondary sexual characteristics, but also

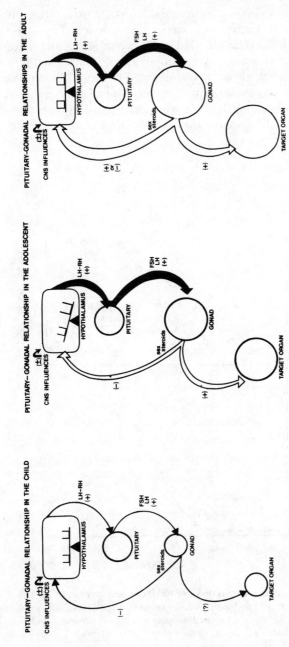

Figure 1-2. A schematic summary of the changes in hypothalamic–pituitary–gonadal interrelationships during postnatal development. The (+) sign indicates stimulation and the (−) sign inhibition. The width of each arrow reflects the secretion rates of gonadotropin-releasing hormone (LH-RH), gonadotropins (FSH and LH), and sex steroids. Reproduced with permission from J. S. D. Winter, C. Faiman, and F. I. Reyes, *Clinical Obstetrics and Gynecology*, **21**, 71 (1978).

modulate the relative amounts of FSH and LH secreted by the pituitary. In girls, the ovarian cycle of sequential follicular maturation and atresia imposes a rhythmic pattern on estrogen production (Figure 1-5), which in time leads to menarche, the first endometrial sloughing. After several months of such anovular cycles an ovarian follicle finally produces sufficient estradiol to elicit a preovulatory LH surge. The appearance of ovulatory menstrual cycles is a relatively late phenomenon of female puberty. There is much less information regarding the development of male fertility, but spermatozoa usually appear in the urine by mid-puberty.

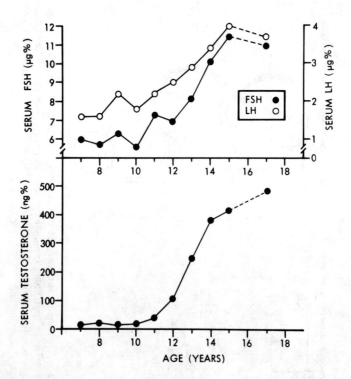

Figure 1-3. Mean serum concentrations of FSH, LH, and testosterone obtained during a mixed longitudinal study of 56 healthy adolescent boys. Reproduced with permission from C. Faiman and J. S. D. Winter, "Gonadotropins and Sex Hormone Patterns in Puberty: Clinical Data", in M. M. Grumbach, G. D. Grave, and F. E. Mayer, *Control of the Onset of Puberty,* Wiley, New York, 1974, p. 39.

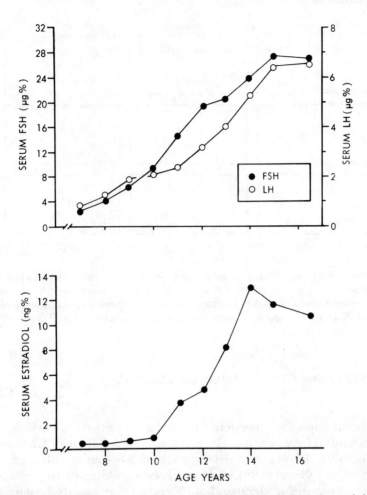

Figure 1-4. Mean serum concentrations of FSH, LH, and estradiol observed during a mixed longitudinal study of 58 adolescent girls. Reproduced with permission from C. Faiman and J.S.D. Winter, "Gonadotropins and Sex Hormone Patterns in Puberty: Clinical Data," in M. M. Grumbach, G. D. Grave, and F. E. Mayer, *Control of the Onset of Puberty,* Wiley, New York, 1974, p. 46.

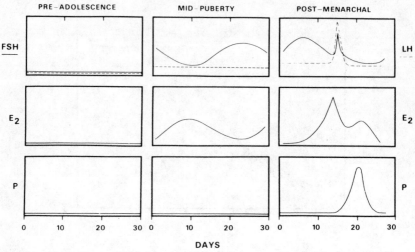

Figure 1-5. A schematic summary of the changes in both serum concentrations and rhythmic secretion patterns of FSH, LH, estradiol (E_2), and progesterone (P) which mark the development of adult ovulatory menstrual cycles. Reproduced with permission from C. Faiman, J. S. D. Winter, and F. I. Reyes, *Clinical Obstetrics and Gynecology,* **3,** 467 (1976).

THE INFLUENCE OF NUTRITION ON PUBERTY

The clinical impact of disordered nutrition on puberty is obvious, but the mechanism by which this effect is achieved is less clear. Childhood undernutrition delays sexual development, in association with a general slowing of growth and maturation (8). In obese children neuroendocrine maturation may be accelerated, but this effect may be offset somewhat by reduced gonadal responsiveness to gonadotropic stimulation. Frisch and Revelle (9) observed a similar average body weight at menarche in early- and late-maturing girls and suggested that the timing of puberty might be related to the acquisition of some critical weight or percentage body fat. Frisch (10) has postulated that pubertal adipose tissue is directly involved in the programming of adolescent maturation through its ability to metabolize sex steroids and thus influence the production of estrogens. This hypothesis has found little experimental support, however, and most endocrinologists would suggest instead that sexual maturation and body fat accumulation are parallel but unrelated processes, both of which are influenced by nutrition and growth rate (11).

There is obvious teleological merit in maintaining a close relationship of sexual maturation to nutrition, by a mechanism such as changing hypothalamic metabolism of catecholamines, endorphins, or other neurotransmitters. There is an obvious analogy between such a mechanism in puberty and that by which seasonal-breeding species regulate the pattern of pulsatile GnRH secretion so as to ensure delivery of offspring when food is plentiful (12, 13).

This relationship has been studied most extensively in patients with amenorrhea secondary to anorexia nervosa (14). These patients show gonadotropin levels, secretory patterns, and responses to exogenous GnRH which resemble those of normal prepubertal girls. In addition they may show partial diabetes insipidus and abnormalities in thermoregulation and catecholamine metabolism which suggest a derangement in hypothalamic aminergic neurotransmission. Administration of a low-dose pulsatile infusion of GnRH for 5 days to such patients elicits changes in FSH and LH secretion similar to those seen during early puberty (15). A similar transition, with eventual resumption of the adult pattern of gonadotropin secretion, occurs following satisfactory weight gain.

It seems clear that most of these phenomena are a result of starvation, although in anorexia nervosa additional psychologic factors may perturb hypothalamic function. Delayed puberty or secondary amenorrhea has also been observed in female athletes and ballet dancers, suggesting that not only the level of food intake but also other factors such as physical activity and competition may influence reproductive function (16). Indeed in amenorrheic ballet dancers a short period of forced inactivity may permit a resumption of menses without any obvious change in body weight.

This chapter demonstrates that puberty is not an event, but a logical sequence of maturational processes that eventually produce adult reproductive function. Of central importance in its timing is an as yet only partially understood mechanism whereby pulsatile secretion of hypothalamic GnRH is inhibited throughout childhood, thus permitting a decade of parental nurturing that certainly has been critical to the social evolution of man. The duration of this inhibition, and thus of childhood itself, can be affected by various external factors, one of the most important of which is the level of nutrition. Studies of patients with anorexia nervosa indicate that puberty is not a one-way process, but can be reversed by malnutrition, possibly in a manner similar to that operative in seasonal-breeding animals.

REFERENCES

1. J. S. D. Winter, C. Faiman, and F. I. Reyes, "Sex Steroid Production by the Human Fetus: Its Role in Morphogenesis and Control by Gonadotropins," in *Morphogenesis and Malformation of the Genital System,* Alan R. Liss, New York, 1977, pp. 41–58.

2. J. A. Clements, F. I. Reyes, J. S. D. Winter, and C. Faiman, *Proc. Soc. Exp. Biol. Med.,* **163,** 437 (1980).

3. J. S. D. Winter, C. Faiman, W. C. Hobson, A. V. Prasad, and F. I. Reyes, *J. Clin. Endocrinol. Metab.,* **40,** 545 (1975).

4. J. S. D. Winter and C. Faiman, *J. Clin. Endocrinol. Metab.,* **35,** 561 (1972).

5. D. C. Anderson, *Lancet,* **2,** 454 (1980).

6. R. M. Boyar, J. W. Finkelstein, H. Roffway, S. Kapen, E. D. Weitzman, and L. Hellman, *New Engl. J. Med.,* **287,** 528 (1972).

7. C. Faiman and J. S. D. Winter, "Gonadotropin and Sex Hormone Patterns in Puberty: Clinical Data," in M. M. Grumbach, G. D. Grave, and F. E. Mayer, Eds.. *Control of the Onset of Puberty,* Wiley, New York, 1974, pp. 32–61.

8. S. Dreizen, C. N. Spirakis, and R. E. Stone, *J. Pediat.,* **70,** 256 (1967).

9. R. E. Frisch and R. Revelle, *Science,* **169,** 397 (1970).

10. R. E. Frisch, *Federation Proc.,* **39,** 2395 (1980).

11. A. R. Glass and R. S. Swerdloff, *Federation Proc.,* **39,** 2360 (1980).

12. G. A. Lincoln, *J. Endocr.,* **83,** 251 (1979).

13. L. Wildt, G. Marshall, and E. Knobil, *Science,* **207,** 1373 (1980).

14. R. A. Vigersky, *Anorexia Nervosa,* Raven Press, New York, 1977.

15. J. C. Marshall and R. P. Kelch, *J. Clin. Endocrinol. Metab.,* **49,** 712 (1979).

16. R. E. Frisch, G. Wyshak, and L. Vincent, *New Engl. J. Med.,* **303,** 17 (1980).

2

Changes in Body Composition during Adolescence

JO ANNE BRASEL, M.D.

UCLA School of Medicine and Harbor-UCLA Medical Center, Torrance, California

The growth rate during adolescence is greater than any other time of postnatal life except for the first year of life. At the end of the 5-year adolescent period the gain in weight in both sexes is 65% of initial weight, or stated differently, 40% of final weight. In essence, total body weight is not quite doubled in this period. Height gains account for approximately 15% of adult height. This phenomenal growth requires a great increase in nutrient intake and makes the period particularly vulnerable for nutritional imbalances. This chapter will describe the composition of this growth, particularly as it differs between the sexes, and will present, at least briefly, current concepts regarding the hormonal factors responsible for these changes.

In healthy, well-nourished children body composition before puberty is essentially similar in the two sexes, although females are noted to have slightly more subcutaneous fat than males from birth on. During the middle childhood years body fat is approximately 18% of total body weight. The remainder (82%) is lean body mass. By young adulthood (18 years) male body fatness has decreased slightly to approximately 15% and female fatness has increased significantly to approximately 28%. Therefore lean body mass is 85% of weight in young adult males and 72% in females. Using these percentages and data on mean weight of United States subjects collected by the National Center for Health Statistics, one can estimate absolute amounts of body fat and lean body mass in the two sexes. The average 18-year-old male weighing 68.9 kg contains 10.3 kg of fat and 58.6 kg of lean tissue. The figures for an 18-year-old female weighing 56.6 kg are 15.8 kg of fat and 40.8 kg of lean tissue. These significant, hormonally determined differences persist throughout adulthood even as both sexes increase the percent body fat with advancing age.

These data have provided an overall view of adolescent growth. Let us reexamine this period of remarkable growth in somewhat more detail. The sexes require examination separately not only because of body composition differences, but also because of differences in the timing of puberty. On average girls enter and complete puberty 2 years earlier than boys.

Growth rates are very high in the first two years, approximately 10 inches per year, but fall off rapidly to rates of 2 to 3 inches per year between 3 and 10 years of age. Just after 10 years the average girl enters the adolescent growth spurt and the growth rate rises to reach a peak and then falls to zero as growth ceases because of fusion of the epiphyseal centers. The age of peak height velocity varies from 10.2 years for early maturers to 13.8 years for late maturers, with the average age being 12 years. The onset of the growth spurt is 8 years for early maturers, 11.5 years for late maturers, and 10 years on average. At the peak the height gained ranges from 3 to 3½ inches per year on average for the three groups, but can be as great as 4.4 inches for rapidly growing early maturers to as little as 2.2 inches for slow growing late maturers. Growth is essentially over by 15 years in the average girl. In the five years of adolescence, that is, from 10 to 15 years, the average girl grows 9¼ inches and gains 46 pounds.

In boys the general shape of the growth rate curve is similar but the adolescent spurt occurs 2 years later. Age of peak velocity is at 12.2, 14.0, and 15.8 years for early, average, and late maturers, respectively. The age of onset ranges from 9.5 to 13.5 years, with an average of 12 years. Peak height velocity ranges from 5.1 to 2.2 inches per year and averages 3.7. Growth ceases at approximately 17 years of age. In the five years of adolescence, that is, from 12 to 17 years, the average boy grows 10.4 inches and gains 58 pounds. Thus men are taller and heavier than women for two reasons: they grow for a longer period of time and they also grow slightly more during adolescence.

Similar curves have been developed for weight velocity which are identical in shape. In boys peak weight velocity occurs at the same age as peak height velocity, whereas it is slightly later (approximately 6 months) in girls.

How is this growth packaged? I noted earlier that during adolescence girls deposit relatively more total body fat and boys more lean tissue.

Subcutaneous fat, as measured by skinfold thickness, participates in that process. It is rapidly deposited in the first few months postnatally; by 4 to 6 months of age the rate of deposition slows, and by 1 year of age skinfold thickness actually begins to decline as children lose their "baby fat." At 8 years of age this trend is reversed and the relentless battle of the bulge begins for females. The rate of increase in subcutaneous fat is even steeper after 13 years, the approximate age of the first menstrual period. This is in distinct contrast to the pattern of subcutaneous fat deposition during adolescence in boys. The pattern in boys in early life is similar to that in girls. There is also a preadolescent rise in subcutaneous fat in boys, which begins at 8 years of age and continues until 12 years. But then the patterns diverge and boys actually become leaner during their rapid growth phase. As adolescence ends, however, similar to girls, fat deposition again increases in males. Thus during the middle years both sexes tend to become fatter.

Growth in lean tissue has been documented by measuring total body water or total body potassium, since these constituents are located almost entirely in lean tissue and are virtually absent from adipose tissue. All such studies reveal that early in life the sexes contain similar amounts of lean tissue for body size but during adolescence a difference develops. Beginning at age 13 years it is clear that the amount of lean body mass gained per unit height increases over earlier childhood values in boys and by contrast begins to level off in girls. The major tissue contributing to this lean tissue growth is muscle. Again the major sex difference is seen to be a continued growth in muscle in boys after the time such accumulation ceases in girls. Skeletal growth also continues for a longer time in males and contributes to the total lean tissue discrepancy in adulthood.

What are the hormonal changes that precede and/or accompany these changes in body composition and do they provide any insight into the mechanisms involved? That these changes are hormonally determined seems clear, since studies in man and animals have shown that castration prior to puberty results in an individual whose adult body composition is somewhere between that of the adult male and the adult female unless gender-appropriate hormonal replacement is given at the usual age of puberty.

A number of cross-sectional studies of the hormonal changes of adolescence have been carried out. The signal for the initiation of puberty remains unclear, although studies of large population groups suggest that reaching a certain body size may play some role in this process. This remains a controversial issue. Several events occur before there are any outward manifestations of puberty. These include increased secretory activity of the adrenal cortex and decreased sensitivity of the hypothalamic centers to sex steroids, with consequent increased stimulation of the pituitary to release its gonadal stimulating hormones. Clearly the first pituitary gonadotropin to increase is FSH. These early changes prepare or "prime" the testis or ovary to respond to its subsquent further stimulation. As this stimulation proceeds, sex steroids more biologically active than those of the adrenal are secreted by the gonads and the overt changes of puberty as we know them begin to appear. Early breast development is noted in the female and the external genitalia begin to enlarge in the male. Both sexes then rapidly progress through the accelerated growth phase and full development of secondary sexual characteristics, which is the phase of adolescence that most alters nutrient requirements.

Many questions remain to be answered about puberty, especially those related to the factors that initiate it. Nutritional status prior to puberty as it affects overall growth may well be important in this regard. Additionally it is clear that adequate nutrient intake is necessary if the growth associated with puberty is to be accomplished. It is possible to calculate roughly the approximate caloric value of the tissue deposited. In females the 5-year adolescent growth consists of 9 kg of fat and 12 kg of lean body mass, with caloric values of 81,000 calories and 48,000 calories, respectively. In males the figures are 3 kg of fat and 23 kg of lean body mass, or 27,000 calories and 92,000 calories, respectively. These calculations include nothing for the digestion, absorption, or deposition of those calories, which would, of course, increase the energy cost of adolescent growth even further. Hence it is not surprising that decreased energy availability significantly affects adolescent growth and that achievement of full growth potential during this critical period of development is dependent upon adequate nutrient intake.

SUGGESTED READINGS

Although some of the following papers represent original publications presenting new original data, most are review papers that contain extensive references to original papers in the field. Thus this is not an exhaustive bibliography.

H. V. Barnes, Physical Growth and Development During Puberty, *Med. Clin. N. Am.*, **59**, 1305 (1975).

D. B. Cheek, "Body Compositon, Hormones, Nutrition, and Adolescent Growth," in M. M. Grumbach, G. D. Grave, and F. E. Mayer, Eds., *The Control of the Onset of Puberty*, Wiley, New York, 1974, pp. 424–442.

C. Faiman and J. S. D. Winter, "Gonadotropins and Sex Hormone Patterns in Puberty: Clinical Data," in M. M. Grumbach, G. D. Grave, and F. E. Mayer, Eds., *The Control of the Onset of Puberty*, Wiley, New York, 1974, pp. 32–35.

G. B. Forbes, "Biological Implications of the Adolescent Growth Process: Body Composition," in J. I. McKigney and H. N. Munro, Eds., *Nutrient Requirements in Adolescence*, MIT Press, Cambridge, 1976, pp. 57–66.

M. G. Forest, E. De Peretti, and J. Bertrand, Hypothalamic–Pituitary–Gonadal Relationships in Man from Birth to Puberty, *Clin. Endocrinol.*, **5**, 551 (1976).

B. Friis-Hansen, "Hydrometry of Growth and Aging," in J. Brozek, Ed., *Human Body Composition*, Pergamon, Oxford, 1965, pp. 191–209.

R. E. Frisch, "Critical Weight at Menarche, Initiation of the Adolescent Growth Spurt, and Control of Puberty," in M. M. Grumbach, G. D. Grave, and F. E. Mayer, Eds., *The Control of Onset of Puberty*, Wiley, New York, 1974, pp. 403–423.

M. M. Grumbach, J. C. Roth, S. L. Kaplan, and R. P. Kelch, "Hypothalamic–Pituitary Regulation of Puberty in Man: Evidence and Concepts Derived from Clinical Research," in M. M. Grumbach, G. D. Grave, and F. E. Mayer, Eds., *The Control of the Onset of Puberty*, Wiley, New York, 1974, pp. 115–166.

A. Häger, L. Sjöstrom, B. Arivdsson, P. Björntorp, and U. Smith, Body Fat and Adipose Tissue Cellularity in Infants: A Longitudinal Study, *Metab.*, **26**, 607 (1977).

F. E. Johnston, A. F. Roche, L. M. Schnell, and N. B. Wettenhall, Critical Weight at Menarche. Critique of a Hypothesis, *Am. J. Dis. Child.*, **129**, 19 (1975).

W. A. Marshall, Growth and Sexual Maturation in Normal Puberty, *Clin. Endocrinol. Metab.*, **4**, 3 (1975).

E. D. Mellits and D. B. Cheek, The Assessment of Body Water and Fatness from Infancy to Adulthood, *Mongr. Soc. Res. Child. Develop.*, **35**, 7 (1970).

A. Parra, C. Cervantes, M. Sanchez, L. Fletes, G. Garcia-Bulness, R. M. Argote, A. Carranco, I. Sojo, and V. Cortes-Gallegos, The Relationship of Plasma Gonadotropins and Androgen Concentrations to Body Growth in Boys, *Acta Endocrinol. (Kbh)*, in press.

A. Parra, C. Cervantes, M. Sanchez, L. Fletes, G. Garcia-Bulness, R. M. Argote, I. Sojo, A. Carranco, R. Arias, and V. Cortes-Gallegos, The Relationship of Plasma Gonadotropins and Steroid Concentrations to Body Growth in Girls, *Acta Endocrinol. (Kbh)*, in press.

R. F. Pierson, Jr., D. H. Y. Lin, and R. A. Phillips, Total Body Potassium in Health: Effects of Age, Sex, Height, and Fat, *Am. J. Physiol.*, **226**, 206 (1974).

E. O. Reiter and A. W. Root, Hormonal Changes of Adolescence, *Med. Clin. N. Am.*, **59**, 1289 (1975).

K. Schlüter, W. Funfack, J. Pachaly, and B. Weber, Development of Subcutaneous Fat in Infancy. Standards for Tricipital, Subscapular, and Suprailiacal Skinfolds in German Infants, *Europ. J. Pediat.*, **132**, 255 (1976).

J. M. Tanner, *Growth at Adolescence*, 2nd Ed., Blackwell, Oxford, 1962.

J. M. Tanner and R. H. Whitehouse, Clinical Longitudinal Standards for Height, Weight, Height Velocity, Weight Velocity, and the Stages of Puberty, *Arch. Dis. Child.*, **51**, 170 (1976).

J. M. Tanner and R. H. Whitehouse, Revised Standards for Triceps and Subscapular Skinfolds in British Children, *Arch. Dis. Child.*, **50**, 142 (1975).

J. M. Tanner, R. H. Whitehouse, E. Marubini, and L. F. Resele, The Adolescent Growth Spurt of Boys and Girls of the Harpenden Growth Study, *Ann. Hum. Biol.*, **3**, 109 (1976).

L. Zacharias and R. J. Wurtman, Age at Menarche. Genetic and Environmental Influences, *N. Engl. J. Med.*, **280**, 868 (1969).

3

Nutritional Requirements of Adolescents

WILLIAM A. DANIEL, JR., M.D.

University of Alabama School of Medicine, Birmingham, Alabama

Adolescence is the only period of life after birth in which the velocity of growth accelerates. The dramatic physical changes of the body include increases in height and weight, deposition and redistribution of fat, increased lean body mass, and enlargement of many organs, including the sexual components whereby the adolescent can beget or conceive. It is obvious that nutrition is closely related to these physical changes and, as in infancy, optimal nutrition is necessary for optimal growth. It is surprising that little nutrition research has been concerned with normal growth during adolescence. Nutrition surveys have included adolescents and results are presented in various chronologic groupings, although we all recognize the tremendous variation in the time of onset of puberty, the different velocity of growth, and the length of time required to achieve adult stature. Because menarche is an objective milestone of female adolescent growth, it has been used in nutritional studies, but there has been no general maturational counterpart for boys. Any group of young adolescents is likely to consist of boys and girls of greatly differing stature and weight with some still young children and others almost adult in size. Chronologic age is a poor reference point for the study of adolescents.

Many methods have been used to assess growth. Height and weight have been used for centuries. Skinfold thickness has been added by nutritionists. Eruption of specific teeth contributes to the judging of the stage of maturation. The most accurate means of evaluating where a particular adolescent boy or girl is along the maturational curve at a particular time is the use of skeletal age. However, radiographs are often unavailable, can be expensive, or may be contraindicated. Studies of growth at adolescence began many decades ago and these were reviewed by Tanner who, using his mixed longitudinal studies, developed a classification of maturity based on changes in secondary sex characteristics (1). These changes have high concordance with skeletal age and have been found to be of great value in assessing growth of individual adolescents.

SEX MATURITY RATINGS (SMR)

Tanner's system of rating stages of maturity is based on changes of the breasts and pattern of pubic hair in girls and on changes in genitalia and in pubic hair pattern in boys. In each sex, the observer rates pubic hair pattern and breast or genital changes separately; if a single rating is desired, the mean value of the two ratings is used. Rating 1 is prepubertal and rating 5, for practical purposes, is adult, although there is usually some physical growth after this rating is reached. Characteristics for the five ratings are given in Table 3-1.

A few general associations should be remembered. The peak height velocity for girls occurs most often between pubic hair rating 2 and breast rating 3; for boys, the peak height velocity is between pubic hair ratings 3 and 4 (2). Menarche occurs most often at SMR 4 for pubic hair and breasts, although some girls begin menstruation at an earlier stage of maturity. There are associated changes in both sexes which are more easily observed by nutritionists. For example, axillary hair usually first appears when pubic hair is just reaching rating 4, although this is variable. About the same time, boys begin to develop facial hair, which begins to increase in length and pigmentation at the corners of the upper lip and, with time, spreads medially to form a faint mustache. Hair also begins to appear on the arms and legs and continues to grow in length and becomes darker with age. At the time of axillary hair growth, the apocrine sweat glands of the axilla enlarge and produce a recognizable, characteristic odor. These changes in boys, and menarche in girls, give an approximate indication of the stage of maturity. If a girl has not begun to menstruate, it is likely that the SMR is 3, provided the height and weight show she has had a spurt of growth. Frisch (3) reports that both black and white girls must have a weight of approximately 46 kg for menarche to occur, although some girls of very small stature will

Table 3-1. Sex Maturity Ratings[a]

		Boys	
Stage	Pubic Hair	Penis	Testes
1	None	Preadolescent	Predolescent
2	Scanty, long, slightly pigmented	Slight enlargement	Enlarged scrotum, pink texture altered
3	Darker, starts to curl, small amount	Penis longer	Larger
4	Resembles adult type, but less in quantity; coarse, curly	Larger; glans and breadth increase in size	Larger, scrotum dark
5	Adult distribution, spread to medial surface of thighs	Adult	Adult

		Girls	
Stage	Pubic Hair	Breasts	
1	Preadolescent	Preadolescent	
2	Sparse, lightly pigmented straight, medial border of labia	Breast and papilla elevated as small mound; areolar diameter increased	
3	Darker, beginning to curl, increased amount	Breast and areola enlarged, no contour separation	
4	Coarse, curly, abundant, but amount less than in adult	Areola and papilla form secondary mound	
5	Adult feminine triangle spread to medial surface of thighs	Mature; nipple projects, areola part of general breast contour	

[a] Adapted from J. M. Tanner, *Growth of Adolescence*, 2nd. ed, Blackwell, Oxford, 1962.

weigh less. If menstruation has occurred, the nutritionist can assume the girl is at SMR 4, that growth is decelerating and fewer calories are needed. In a boy, the absence of axillary and extremity hair, or change in the voice, indicates in general that development is less than rating 4 and this rating can be closely correlated with height and weight changes.

With practice, sex maturity ratings are easily estimated, and if such estimates can be compared with those obtained by physical examination, one's skill rapidly increases. For readers who wish more detailed information about growth at adolescence Tanner's classic text is available (1). Adolescence is characterized by cognitive and psychosocial growth in addition to physical changes and all three of these areas of change can affect nutrition in adolescence.

COGNITIVE AND PSYCHOSOCIAL GROWTH

Most children think in concrete terms at the onset of puberty. That is, they think in terms based upon past and present experiences. They cannot fully appreciate the future, form hypotheses, or pursue abstract thought in arriving at logical conclusions. With adolescence, most normal children begin to change in cognitive development and gradually develop formal operational thought. This process enables the individual to consider a variety of possibilities, to project these options to future relationships and consequences, and, although past experiences still play a role in thinking, they are tempered and altered by hypothetical consideration.

During adolescence, boys and girls begin to move in a wider geographic area and to encounter situations not previously experienced. They must begin the process of separation from the family; that is, not only physical separation but emotional distancing coupled with the assumption of responsibility for oneself. As they become older, they are more and more aware of the need for vocational training or preparation for a vocation by further education; they realize that they must become self-supporting, and they usually want to work to obtain material goods. Early adolescence is also characterized by development of the sexual anatomical parts, awareness of sexual thoughts and desires, the need to establish personal moral codes and to learn how one copes with being male or female in a particular society and group. Growth in these three large areas—physical, cognitive, and psychosocial—is not necessarily synchronous and there is often a temporary or permanent disequilibrium that can affect overall adolescent development.

It is obvious, for example, that early physical growth unassociated with the development of formal operational thought may, for example, lead to pregnancy without awareness of the need for adequate nutrition. If a very young pregnant girl cannot appreciate the future, cannot think abstractly about the needs of the infant she will bear or the need for appropriate prenatal care, surely her nutritional status will suffer. And nutritional counseling appropriate for a female who is farther along in cognitive growth will not be understood by the younger girl. Nutritional counseling of early adolescents must be in simple terms, related to past and present experiences when possible, or to recognizable examples; and education must be repeated and expanded with the changes in the adolescent's cognitive growth. We have found that the most effective acceptance of nutritional counseling occurs when the patient likes the nutritionist and wishes to please her. Some early adolescents are capable of a degree of formal operational thought, and counseling must be correlated with the stage of development, for talking too simply to a highly intellectual adolescent will bring about rejection of the advice. Unfortunately, there are no simple, easily performed, reliable tests to use for cognitive stages of growth, but conversing with an adolescent will give clues to the level of thinking.

Sickle cell disease, for example, is often associated with delayed puberty and growth. It is therefore desirable that nutritionists providing care of adolescents evaluate their client's progress physically, cognitively, and psychosocially, even though nutrition counseling has been and is primarily related to physical growth. This chapter stresses the relationship of physical growth to normal nutrition in adolescents, for it has been found that many such relationships are statistically more concordant with sex maturity ratings than with chronologic age. In the discussion that follows, data are from our own studies of normal, healthy adolescents seen in an adolescent clinic for children of low income families. Some of the data were compared with findings from adolescent girls of upper middle income families. Caloric intake, iron intake, hematocrits, alkaline phosphatase, and folate determinations will be presented.

CALORIC INTAKE

The stereotypic picture of an adolescent boy is a thin young man who is always hungry and always eating. We usually do not think of adolescent girls in this manner. It has been shown that girls mature about 1½ to 2 years earlier than boys and each sex has a dramatic growth spurt. We may ask whether adolescent girls and boys of the same age have different caloric intakes and, if in general boys grow taller than girls, do they have greater caloric intakes at the time of peak height velocity? We found a very great range in the number of calories consumed by boys and girls of both races at all sex maturity ratings. Our findings showed that girls had their highest caloric intake at mean SMR 2, the time of peak height velocity. Low income white girls did eat more at SMR 4, but with that one exception, all girls, regardless of income or race, decreased their caloric intakes after the peak height velocity, regardless of increasing maturity. Boys, on the other hand, continued to consume more calories as they became more mature, and white boys ate more than black boys, according to mean caloric intakes. Boys consistently took in more calories than girls (Figure 3-1) except for white boys at SMR 2.

Recommended Dietary Allowance (RDA) values for boys 11–14 years of age are 2700 kcal and 2800 kcal for 15–18 years. In our population, mean caloric intake for boys showed a steady rise from 2400 kcal at age

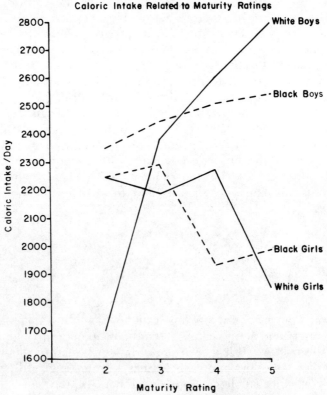

Figure 3-1.   Dietary intake correlated with maturity ratings.

12 years to 2900 kcal at 17 years. The RDA for girls 11–14 years of age is 2200 kcal and 2100 kcal for 15–18 years. Girls in our study consumed 2500 kcal at 12 years and decreased to 1950 kcal by age 17 years. Statistical correlation of caloric intake is greater with sex maturity ratings than with chronologic age.

DIETARY IRON INTAKE

The mean iron intake of each study subject, calculated from the 24-hour recall, was computed and graphed according to race–sex categories at each sex maturity rating and according to chronologic age. When the mean iron intakes were related to SMRs, males and females of each race had comparable intakes at rating 2, the first visible signs of pubescence. There was a sharp increase in the intake of white subjects, particularly males, and this continued throughout the stages of increasing maturity. The same trend was present in black males. Intakes for white girls increased through adolescence, with the exception of a decrease at SMR 4. The intakes for male adolescents were significantly larger than those for adolescent females at all sex maturity ratings except SMR 2.

The RDA for dietary iron for children older than 11 years of age is 18 mg. None of the mean iron intakes of any of the groups of our subjects met this RDA (Figure 3-2). White subjects had higher mean intakes at all sex maturity ratings than black adolescents. It is interesting that there

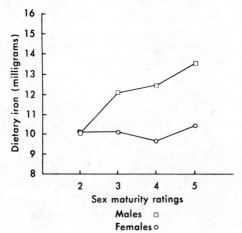

Figure 3-2. Iron intake for adolescents related to maturity, sex, and race.

was no significant difference between the mean iron intakes of girls from low and high income families. It is also important to note that mean iron intakes for black adolescents were lower than, but roughly parallel to, the mean intakes for white subjects.

Hematocrits

Hematocrit determinations were obtained from 1007 adolescent girls and 1000 adolescent boys who were judged to be healthy. Statistical relationships were determined using sex−race−SMR and sex−race−age, and there was higher concordance with sex maturity ratings than with age. As is evident in Figure 3-3, there was little change in hematocrit percentages as girls became more mature. The value of SMR 1 for white girls is probably too high and represents a stage of growth in which puberty had started but was not evident to us on physical examination. Figure 3-4 illustrates the rise in hematocrit percentages for adolescent boys related to increasing maturity and it is assumed that increased hematocrit percentages are related to the increasing testosterone stimulus on the bone marrow; thus boys have higher hematocrit and

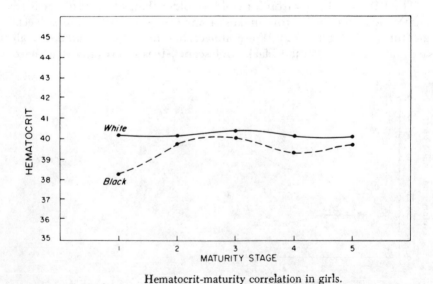

Hematocrit-maturity correlation in girls.

Figure 3-3.   Hematocrit values correlated with sex, race, and sex maturity ratings as shown in girls.

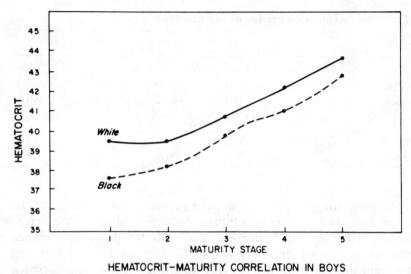

Figure 3-4.   Hematocrit values correlated with sex, race, and sex maturity ratings as shown in boys.

hemoglobin values than girls. It is also evident from these figures that black subjects had lower hematocrit percentages than white subjects at all SMRs (4).

Anemia

In our study population, we used the 15th percentile below the mean as the criterion for diagnosing anemia and these values were related to sex, race, and sex maturity ratings. Garn and Smith (5) have shown that blacks have approximately 1 g less hemoglobin than whites and this is unrelated to diet, income level, education, or age. Therefore different standards are used in screening for anemia in our adolescent subjects.

With these standards (Table 3-2) adolescents were identified as possibly having anemia. In those subjects with anemia, transferrin saturation was calculated as an indicator of body iron stores. Serum ferritin determinations may be a more accurate indicator, but this procedure was not available when the study was begun. A transferrin saturation percentage at or below 16 was used to indicate inadequate stores of iron. In girls, 2.5% were found to have low hematocrits and transferrin saturation below 16% and were classified as anemic.

Table 3-2.   15th Percentiles of Hematocrits

SMR	1	2	3	4	5
			Males		
White	35.6	36.9	38.2	39.6	40.9
Black	34.9	36.0	37.1	38.2	39.3
			Females		
White	35.8	36.6	37.0	36.7	35.9
Black	34.0	35.3	36.0	36.2	35.8

An interesting finding was present in our adolescent boys, 22.3% of whom had low hematocrits, a figure similar to findings of the Ten State Nutrition Survey (6). Using our standards for diagnosing suspected anemia, it seemed strange that this finding would be 9 times more frequent in boys than in girls. In comparing the low hematocrits with percentages of transferrin saturation, 85% of the "anemia" group had transferrin saturation values greater than 20%; in fact, most percentages were above 30. Only 3.3% of all boys had low hematocrit and low transferrin saturation percentages, our criterion for diagnosing anemia. This figure is only slightly greater than the 2.5% for girls.

It was then found that the boys having low hematocrits with normal or high transferrin saturation were maturationally between mean SMR 3 and 4, as shown in Figure 3-5. This is the period of peak height velocity which in a few months is followed by significant increase in lean body mass in boys. Plasma volume also rises more in the male than in the female (1) and other changes in body fluid compartments, tissues, quantity of fat, number of erythrocytes, and so on occur and apparently bring about sex differences. We assume, but have not proved, that increased plasma volume dilutes the hemoglobin mass, thus giving lower unit measurements. It is also likely that the oxygen supply at the cellular level is adequate for normal physiologic function. Another point of conjecture

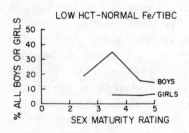

Figure 3-5. Percentage of adolescents having low hematocrits and normal transferrin saturation correlated with sex maturing rating.

is the relationship of increasing testosterone concentration in males and the relationship of 2,3-diphosphoglycerate. To our knowledge there are no data for concentrations of 2,3-DPG in adolescence or of values related to sex maturity ratings. With increased velocity of growth, one can hypothesize that the concentration of 2,3-DPG slightly increases and thus provides a greater shift to the right in the hemoglobin—oxygen dissociation curve to provide adequate oxygen to the tissues. These possibilities remain to be tested.

Administering iron to several of the boys having low hematocrits with high transferrin saturation produced no change in hematocrit percentages. But, in boys with these findings, there was most often a return to normal hematocrit values when growth had reached a higher ordinal sex maturity rating. In our adolescent clinic, we believe it is necessary to obtain serum ferritin values or percentages of transferrin saturation in boys having low hematocrit percentages before a diagnosis of anemia is made.

Another interesting finding in the study was that 14.6% of girls from low income families had hematocrit percentages in the normal range associated with low transferrin saturation percentages. Typically, this group of girls would not be suspected of anemia, but they may represent a high-risk group for developing iron deficiency anemia under conditions of stress.

SERUM ALKALINE PHOSPHATASE

Measurement of serum alkaline phosphatase can serve as an indicator of bone growth. This laboratory test is also related to hepatic function and possible liver disease. The literature carries ranges of alkaline phosphatase for children and adults, but typically does not present it for adolescents, with rare exceptions. It is expected that the growth spurt would be associated with changes in concentration of alkaline phosphatase.

In our studies (Figure 3-6) it is seen that peaks of serum alkaline phosphatase occur at pubic hair maturity rating 2 for girls and at pubic hair rating 3 for boys. Each of these maturity ratings is the time of peak height velocity and illustrates the fact that serum alkaline phosphatase is highest during the peak of the growth spurt. The range of values is very high, particularly in boys, and high concentrations are rarely related to liver disease unless they occur at SMRs indicating greater stages of

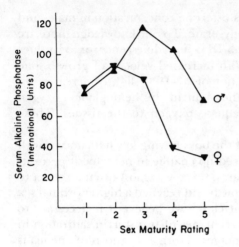

Figure 3-6. The relationship of serum alkalin phosphatase concentrations to sex maturing ratings in adolescents.

maturity. We believe alkaline phosphatase concentrations can add information concerning growth retardation associated with chronic bowel disease or other conditions associated with delayed puberty.

DIETARY INTAKE AND PLASMA CONCENTRATIONS OF FOLATE

With increased growth at adolescence, there is need for folate because of increased cell production. Dietary intake records from our adolescent population were used to calculate the intake of folic acid and correlation was tested using age and sex maturity ratings. Concordance was greater with sex maturity ratings. The results are shown in Figure 3-7 and indicate trends determined by linear regression. It was found that white boys have a significant increase in the intake of folic acid from SMR 2 through SMR 5, indicating that with increasing maturity there is greater intake of folic acid. Black adolescent boys and white adolescent girls had no significant rate of change as they matured. Black girls had a significant decrease in dietary folic acid intake from SMR 2 through SMR 5. Although black subjects had greater intakes at the beginning of puberty, SMR 2, the rapid and greater rate of change of white subjects as they matured indicated that white adolescents had significantly greater intakes of folic acid during late adolescence than blacks. Boys of both races had higher intakes across all maturity ratings than girls of both races.

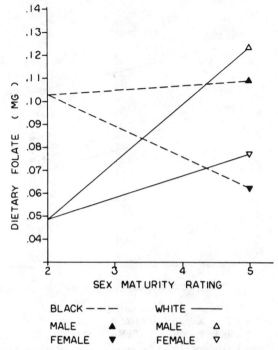

Figure 3-7.   Predicted trends of dietary folate for adolescents.

Figure 3-8, using multiple regression model analysis, shows plasma folate concentrations for both sexes and races. Females had higher plasma concentrations of folate than males across all sex maturity ratings, and all groups had lower plasma folate values as they matured from SMR 2 through SMR 5 ($p<0.0001$).

Increased growth during adolescence implies the need for increased synthesis of purines and pyrimidines for nucleic acid production and the need for increased intake of folic acid. Boys in general double the muscle mass during adolescence, are larger than girls, and one may expect their folate need to be greater. Our data show that boys do have higher intake of dietary folic acid than girls. In the analysis of plasma concentrations of folate, age of the subjects was not a statistically significant factor. Girls had higher concentrations of folate than boys at all sex maturity ratings, the reverse of dietary folic acid intakes. This seemingly paradoxical situation in which boys have higher dietary intakes but lower plasma folate concentrations than girls is thought to represent a greater cellular need for folate in boys. It is our supposition that, although plasma concentrations of folate are lower, with greater disparity in boys between

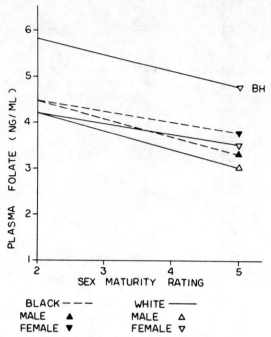

Figure 3-8.   Predicted trends of plasma folate concentrations related to sex, race, and sex maturity ratings of subjects.

intake and plasma values, the tissue and erythropoietic cellular needs are greater in boys, causing a more pronounced negative slope for plasma concentrations when related to sex maturity ratings.

We wish to point out the need for more accurate measurements of folic acid content of foods. Current tables are incomplete and, we believe, often inaccurate, leading to erroneous calculation of dietary folate (7).

PROTEIN

Because adolescence is characterized by rapid physical growth, it is obvious that protein intake should increase to provide the blocks on which adult size can be built. Figure 3-9 presents dietary intake of protein related to sex, race, and sex maturity ratings of the study sample. Correlation with maturity ratings was of higher significance than with chronologic age. The data show that boys of both races had a significant

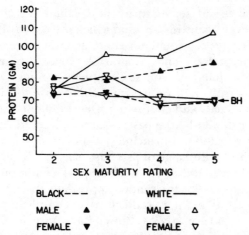

BLACK - - -   WHITE ⎯⎯⎯

MALE ▲   MALE △

FEMALE ▼   FEMALE ▽

Figure 3-9. Daily protein intake correlated with sex maturity ratings, race, and sex.

rate of change as they matured; that is, boys of both races had a positive slope, with white males ($p<0.0003$) having a greater increase of protein intake than black males ($p<0.01$). Black girls in the low economic group also had a significant rate of change with maturity, but white girls in the same economic group did not change significantly as they matured. Boys of both races had a greater intake, rate of change, than girls as they matured from SMR 2 through SMR 5 ($p<0.0001$). Boys had a positive slope, that is, rate of change, whereas girls had a negative slope. As they matured, boys increased their intake of protein and girls decreased the quantity of protein consumed. This finding is in keeping with caloric intake. Also, white adolescent boys had greater protein intake than black boys and the same was true for girls. In Figure 3-9 girls from high income families (BH) show no significant difference in protein intake when compared to that of low income girls. Family income was not a statistically significant factor related to quantity of protein consumed by girls. Mean values for protein intake according to sex, race, and sex maturity ratings were greater than quantities listed by the RDA.

In summary, adolescence is characterized by dramatic changes in physical size and relationship of body parts. Cognitive thought processes and psychosocial growth are integral parts of adolescent growth. These three great areas of change can each exert a reciprocal effect on the others and all must be considered in evaluating the nutritional status of an adolescent and in providing nutritional counseling or management.

In general, nutritional requirements and concentrations of specific nutrients in the blood, as well as other biochemical components, have higher concordance with sex maturity ratings than with chronologic age. There are, however, many instances in which the range of dietary intake of specific nutrients is so wide that neither age nor stage of maturity is a significant factor; for example, vitamin A intake. Nevertheless, nutritionists should be familiar with sex maturity ratings and changes in bodily function at different ratings, and should use this information to judge nutritional needs and counseling. Developmental correlation, not chronologic age, should be the basis of nutrition in adolescence.

In practical application of principles of nutrition in adolescence, how the adolescent thinks, the stage of psychosocial growth, and the presence or absence of chronic illness or handicapping conditions are of great significance. If an adolescent cannot appreciate the need or value of nutritional prescriptions, it is unlikely that compliance will be high. Many adolescents, particularly girls, often have unrealistic views of goals for their bodies and adopt harmful diets without knowing the consequences. Adolescent boys are frequently in error in trying to increase muscle mass or to lose weight in order to qualify for a particular sports category, or they, too, may adopt fad diets related to cult participation. With infants and small children, the nutritionist works with and through the mother. This relationship rarely exists with healthy adolescents and the changes in thinking and psychosocial development are often more significant than they are in young children. It is not enough that the nutritionist be familiar with requirements for adolescent growth; there is also the need to appreciate other aspects of growth related to concepts and actions in early, middle, and late adolescence related to stages of maturity. When this union of information occurs, nutritional service with adolescents can be interesting and rewarding even though there is a great need for further research.

REFERENCES

1. J.M. Tanner, *Growth at Adolescence*, 2nd ed, Blackwell, Oxford, 1962.
2. A.W. Root, *J. Pediat* **83**:1 (1973).
3. R.E. Frisch, *Pediatrics*, **50**(3), 445 (1972).
4. W.A. Daniel, Jr., *Pediatrics*, **52**, 388 (1973).
5. S.M. Garn, J.J. Smith, and D.C. Clark, *J. Nat. Med. Assoc.*, **67**, 91 (1975).
6. Ten-State Nutrition Survey, 1968–1970. IV. Biochemical. DHEW Pub. No. (HSM) 72-8133 (1972).
7. W.A. Daniel, Jr., E.G. Gaines, and D.L. Bennett, *J. Pediatr.*, **86**(2), 288 (1975).

4

Dietary Practices of Adolescents

MAUDENE NELSON, M.S., R.D.

Institute of Human Nutrition, Columbia University College of Physicians and Surgeons, New York, New York

Adolescence is a very dynamic period of life. Particular feelings and needs are evident in the extremes of behavior that characterize the adolescent life-style. Eating behavior is likewise influenced by the attitudes that stem from these feelings (1).

The sense of indestructibility and immortality that is demonstrated by such activities as staying up all night, reckless driving, and drug abuse also results in erratic or poor eating habits. The preoccupation with immediate concerns and the new sense of self-importance mean that the adolescent is understandably shortsighted regarding the long-range benefits and hazards of various eating practices. He or she eats primarily because of hunger. Reducing the consumption of a particular food at this time because of the possibility of hypertension or atherosclerosis later is relatively unimportant. A healthful diet generally has a low priority.

There is a strong need for emotional defenses as the teen emerges from childhood to adulthood. Anorexia nervosa and some cases of obesity are examples of food being used as a defense against an uncomfortable or uncertain reality. In many instances, unconventional or self-styled dietary regimens, such as Zen macrobiotics or vegetarianism, may be behavioral responses through food for the adolescent to identify or isolate him or herself (2–5).

Clearly, each of these needs can result in deleterious nutritious consequences. However, these inferences are not enough to conclude that adolescents are teetering on the edge of malnutrition or that they have no acumen in matters of food and nutrition. In fact, at least 65% of adolescent females are actively involved in shopping for and preparing family food. The adolescent female spends more than one out of four dollars of the family's weekly food expenditure. She exerts her own purchase decisions over brand and variety, and is rapidly emerging as an increasingly better informed consumer (6−8).

NUTRIENTS FOUND TO BE LOW IN ADOLESCENT DIETS

Given the dynamics of this phase of maturation and the assortment of foods in our society, the question of the existence of dietary inadequacies is a valid one. Of the several surveys of adolescent eating patterns conducted in North America many similarities emerge (9−23).

Dietary adequacy is determined by dividing the recommended level of intake by the reported level of consumption. The criterion generally used is that the reported intake for a specific nutrient be at least two-thirds of the Recommended Dietary Allowance (RDA). Nine nutrients from the RDA are used. If less than two-thirds of one nutrient is consumed, the diet is considered poor.*

The nutrients most often found in inadequate amounts are iron (particularly for females), calcium, thiamine, and vitamin A (22, 23, 25). In the Ten-State Nutrition Survey, protein was noted to be low in black and Spanish American females (22). Compared to males, the diets of females contained a greater number of nutrients below the RDA and a larger percentage of the sample showed inadequacies (25).

Instead of RDAs, Haley et al. judged dietary histories against the recommended frequency of consumption from six food catagories. Summarized in Table 4-1, their findings suggest that dietary adequacy (with the exception of meats and breads) declines with age.

Clearly, a significant percentage of adolescents are consuming diets that do not meet the recommended levels of intake for key nutrients.

---

*Because of the periodic revisions of the RDAs this method lends itself to misrepresenting the adequacy of diets in earlier surveys. In one case the percentage of diets that met the RDAs rose from 46 when judged by the 1948 version to 73 when judged by the 1963 version (24).

Table 4-1.   Changes In Adequacy of Diet with Increasing Age[a]

	Age:	10	13	15
		Percent With Adequate Intakes		
Overall diet		54	37	26
Meats		97	82	91
Breads		74	78	77
Milk		74	48	33
Fruit		43	42	31
Vegetables		44	34	38
Cereals		26	33	20

[a]Adapted from Haley et al. (19).

CONSUMPTION PATTERNS

Adolescents are always hungry—or so it seems. Hence, they always seem to be eating. They eat a lot more often than three times a day; up to seven or eight "meals" are common. Because eating is not always in the context of a meal, snacks can and do make significant nutritional contributions. "Regular" eating to a teen may mean approximately the same number of meals and snacks eaten at about the same time each day—not the traditional "3 squares." In addition, a "meal" is defined as whatever food, whether a sandwich or beverage, to which the teen has helped him or herself.

On an average, girls eat more frequently than boys. However, because of sheer volume, teenage boys' diets come much closer than the diets of girls to meeting the recommended level of intake.

According to Huenemann's survey, meal regularity is much more frequent in white and oriental teens than in blacks (the sample included only ten black teens) (18). This survey also found that as meal regularity increased, so too did the nutrient content of the diet. In addition, meal regularity increased with rise in socioeconomic status (SES).

Dinner was the most regularly eaten meal (although black teens tended to omit dinner more often than white teens). Lunch and breakfast were skipped on an average with equal frequency. Breakfast skipping increased as teens got older. Lunches were skipped more during summer months than during the school year. Reasons given for meals skipped included a lack of appetite or time needed to fulfill another commitment (18).

Snacking appeared to pick up the slack of skipped meals and was of particular importance for providing vitamin C. White teenage boys snacked more often than black or oriental boys. The reverse was true for girls. A similar snacking pattern was seen for SES; that is, high SES boys snacked more frequently than black or oriental teens of both sexes (18).

Teens in high SES groups averaged a higher amount of food eaten than teens in middle and low SES groups. Of the actual foods consumed, white teens consumed a greater quantity of dairy, fats, nuts, vegetables, and fruits than oriental or black teens. Black teens lead the group in consumption of desserts and sweets. Oriental teens consumed the highest amount from the grain category—primarily as rice—and a low intake of starchy vegetables. Of the meats and legumes category, orientals also consumed the most among boys and black girls consumed the most among girls. Of the protein foods that were eaten, oriental teens ate more fish than the other two subgroups and black teens ate more pork than the other two subgroups (18).

According to a USDA survey, milk consumption in teenagers has declined. Males from ages 9 to 19 drink only 2½ cups per day and females from ages 9 to 11 consume an average of 2 cups per day. At ages 18 to 19 girls are drinking an average of 1½ cups per day (25).

Soft drink, tea, and coffee consumption is double that of fluid milk in teens' diets. When calories and calcium contributed by dairy foods decrease, soft drinks have usually replaced fluid milk as a beverage at a meal (25).

More raw fruits and vegetables were consumed by girls than by boys, but boys, in turn, consumed the most cooked fruit or juices. Black boys and girls as well as those in the low SES classification ate smaller quantities of raw fruits and vegetables than the other sample subgroups. Black girls tended to be the leading consumers of starchy cooked vegetables (18).

Of the snacks eaten in the Huenemann survey, summarized in Table 4-2, boys seemed to prefer cereals and breads as their first choice and pastry products as their second. Girls, on the other hand, preferred pastry products first and candy second. (Maybe they believed in "sugar and spice and everything nice.")

A 1972 survey of food preferences (15) produced a list of the five most popular foods. In order to deemphasize favorite but infrequent foods, the list was prepared by crossing lists of favorite foods with lists of foods most frequently eaten. In order of preference, the most popular

Table 4-2.   Snack Food Preferences of Boys and Girls (in Descending Order of Popularity)[a]

Boys	Girls
Cereals and bread	Pie, cake, pastry, and cookies
Pie, cake, pastry, and cookies	Candy
Soft drinks	Fruit
Milk	Cereals and bread
Fruit	Soft drinks
Eggs, meat, and cheese	Ice cream

[a]Adapted from Huenemann et al. (18).

foods were soda pop, milk, steak, hamburger, and pizza. The least liked (and least consumed) were liver, fish, squash, clams, and coffee.

A 1971 Gallup Youth Survey of food preferences revealed that some changes are taking place in teens' preferences. See Table 4-3 for a summary. It is interesting that protein foods and ethnic foods have gained popularity over sweets and pastries. But vegetables, a significant source of vitamin A, remain steadfastly unpopular. (There is almost a suggestion that juvenile vagrancy can be controlled by lining the streets with leafy green vegetables.)

Vitamins are consumed by adolescents in significant numbers. In one survey 9 of 51 boys and 22 of 71 girls reported taking vitamins (18). All were from middle or high income classifications. There is a reasonable debate over the issue of whether adolescents should be advised to take supplements. Those teens who would be most likely to benefit from dietary supplements (i.e., lower SES groups) do not seem to be taking

Table 4-3.   Favorite and Least Favorite Foods of Teenagers (in Order of Decreasing Popularity)[a]

Favorite	Least Favorite
Italian foods (e.g., pizza and spaghetti)	Spinach
Steak	Liver
Hamburger	Broccoli
Chicken	Beans
Mexican foods	Squash
Potatoes, French fries	Vegetables (general)

[a]Adapted from the Gallup Youth Survey (21).

any. Furthermore, dietary adequacy should be established before inducing an adolescent to solve an ecological problem with a pill.

SPECIFIC FACTORS THAT INFLUENCE DIETARY PRACTICES

In identifying these areas, the educator and clinician should be better able to provide nutritional support.

Life-Style Complexity

Schorr (15) found that the complexity of life-style had varying significance on nutrient intakes. Although social participation, employment status of teen, fathers' and mothers' occupational levels, and mothers' educational level *were* significant, age, sex, family size, and nutrition information channels *were not*. A factor such as age, although not independently a determinant of food selection, is related to social participation. For example, one must be old enough to make a team, drive a car, and so on. In each of these settings peer group pressure plays an important role in determining who will "give you a break today." Of additional importance was the finding that as the dietary pattern increased in complexity, so, too, did the nutrient intake.

Preferences for Sweet and Salty Tastes

These preferences are very powerful in determining food selection. Karp et al. (11) noted an increased utilization of salty foods as preteen-age black girls increased in age. Another researcher found that the preferences for salty and sweet are distinctly characteristics of age and ethnic groups (26). In this experiment the subjects (N = 618) ages 9 to 15 and 140 adults, were administered four different concentrations of sucrose, lactose, and NaCl. The results, summarized in Table 4-4 are quite striking. Not only did the younger subjects prefer the strongest concentrations but also the young black subjects preferred the strongest solution of NaCl more than any of the other subjects. This presents quite

Table 4-4.   Summary of Preferences for Sweet and Salty in Ages 9–15 and Adults[a]

Concentration of solutions

> young > adult
> adult black > adult white

Sweet concentrations

> young > adult
> young male > young female
> young black > young white

Salty concentrations

> young > adult
> young black > all other groups

[a]Adapted from Desor et al. (26).

a challenge to the clinician who counsels black youth on the reduction of dietary sodium as a preventive measure against hypertension.

Mass Media

Very little evidence is available to show exactly what, if any, effect mass media (primarily television) have on the dietary practices of adolescents. However, if a 5-year-old entering kindergarten has already seen 70,000 30-second advertisements for food (27), that is a monumental amount of questionable nutrition education to be up against. It has been estimated that in a calendar year a teen could watch television for more time than he spends in school. Even if the only dietary practice established as a result of mass media is eating during a commercial, it has an impact on the nutritional well being of the adolescent.

DIETARY PRACTICES OF THE AT-RISK ADOLESCENT

The *obese adolescent* is in a bind. Many clinicians, rather than provide aggressive counseling for weight control, rely on the adolescent growth spurt to use up excess body fat. Anthropometric findings of the HANES survey (28) suggest that the growth spurt does not significantly reduce the amount of excess fat in adolescent females. Concerning intake, several surveys have documented that obese adolescents, in fact, eat less food (fewer calories) than their lean counterparts (16, 17). Overweight teens skip breakfast more often than normal weight teens. Overall, they eat fewer meals and fewer snacks than lean teenagers.

In particular, they eat less food from dairy, vegetable, and fruit groups. Compared to lean teens, overweight teens eat calorically dense foods with much less frequency. As a result of their attempts to eat less, their diets are typically low in iron, calcium, and ascorbic acid.

Obese adolescents are very conscious of their weights. This is particularly true for females. As normal and overweight girls get older a larger percentage of the group view themselves as fat. In contrast, males begin to perceive themselves as thinner as they get older (16). Having observed adolescents in recreational settings, I find it interesting that the males, after a game of basketball, for example, are drinking cartons of orange juice. The females, on the other hand, are sipping no-calorie colas. This practice, although undocumented, is very compatible with the finding described above.

Perhaps the problem of overweight in adolescence (as in all stages of life) is at the other side of the energy balance. Overweight and obese youths are less active than normal weight or lean youths. In questionnaires, obese teens indicate that they recognize the importance of eating a balanced, low calorie diet, but they underrate the value of exercise and activity in weight control (16). Whether it is a problem of brown fat, insufficient physical activity, or a metabolic quirk, for many it is a phenomenon other than overeating.

The *teenage chronic dieter* is among the 60% of 12th grade girls who are or have been on a reducing diet (28). The erratic starving and uncontrolled refeeding are clearly contraindicated in the precariously balanced adolescent diet. This is an area to which clinicians should give serious attention.

The *pregnant teenager* requires very careful attention to the quality of the diet. Efforts to guide pregnant teens to consume the amount and kind of food we know to be necessary for the optimal outcome of pregnancy will depend very much on whether she has accepted her pregnancy. Because pregnancy and eating well are so tightly linked, it is a time when a certain "shaping" of the adolescent's diet may be possible. But one may first have to overcome concerns with weight gain, nausea (and consequent poor appetite), poor knowledge of proper diet, and social obstacles.

Adolescent athletes, although convinced of the importance of nutrition and the well being of the body, share the same misconceptions as their coaches about training regimens. The biggest offender is the training table meal: a 16-oz steak, a mound of buttered potatoes, and four string beans. We are not training lions. The high amounts of protein and fat are both unnecessary and perhaps taxing (29, 30). In addition, a variety of concoctions, supplements, self-styled health drinks (such as the five raw eggs featured in "Rocky"), and belief in "energy" formulas (such as bee pollen and B-complex) abound. Fasting or gorging to reach a weight classification is both common and unhealthy. Education is important to teach both the teen and the athletic organizer the simple principles of energy balance and the use of appropriate dietary fuels.

The overall picture of the dietary practices of adolescents is characterized by frequent eating; preferences for meat, grain and pastry products, and dairy products; distinctions in preferences and practices between males and females; and distinctions in preferences and practices among different ethnic groups and different SES strata. Although subjective impressions and dietary intake surveys leave questions about the qualitative aspects of some of their diets, growth indicators suggest that our concerns should focus on teens with the least amount of resources.

The key to intervention lies in the fact that the majority of adolescents are autonomous during their waking hours and are, therefore, making almost all of their own food choices. Without question, their choices are influenced by their knowledge of nutrition, what foods are available to them, and what resources they have to secure food (20, 31, 32). Parents and educators should encourage adolescents' views and talents in making decisions about purchasing, preparing, and educating for good nutritional well being.

REFERENCES

1. S. B. Caghan, *Am. J. Nursing,* **75,** 1728 (1975).
2. H. Bruch, *Nutrition Today,* **13,** 5 (1978).
3. W. Daniel, Jr., *Ross Dietetic Currents,* **3,** 15 (1977).
4. R. T. Frankle and F. K. Heussenstamm, *Am. J. Public Health,* **64**(1), 11 (1974).
5. N. J. Bowden, *J. School Health,* **43,** 165 (1973).
6. Triangle Communications, Inc., *Seventeen's Food Survey–1979* (1979).
7. Co-Ed Magazine, *Co-Ed Research Report: Eating and Cooking Habits Survey of Co-Ed Readers,* No. 7911 (April, 1979).

8. American Girl, *Food Survey 1978* (1978).

9. W. N. Harris, *J. School Health,* **40**(6), 323 (1970).

10. J. A. Hruban, *J. School Health,* **47**, 33 (1977).

11. R. J. Karp, et al., *J. National Med. Assoc.,* **72**, 197 (1980).

12. B. Cross, R. O. Herrmann, and R. H. Warland, *J. Am. Dietetic Assoc.* **67**, 131 (1978).

13. N. Schwartz, *J. Am. Dietetic Assoc.,* **66**, 28 (1975).

14. J. L. Greger and G. M. Etnyre, *Am. J. Public Health,* **68**, 70 (1978).

15. B. C. Schorr, D. Sanjur, and E. Erickson, *J. Am. Dietetic Assoc.,* **61**, 415 (1972).

16. N. A. Kaufman, R. Poznanski and K. Guggenheim, *J. Am. Dietetic Assoc.,* **66**, 264 (1965).

17. R. L. Huenemann, *Postgraduate Medicine,* **51**, 99 (May, 1972).

18. R. L. Huenemann, L. Shapiro, M. C. Hampton, and B. W. Mitchel, *J. Am. Dietetic Assoc.,* **53**, 17 (1968).

19. M. Haley, D. Aucoin, and J. Rae, *Canadian J. Public Health,* **68**, 301 (1977).

20. K. L. Clancy, B. G. Bibby, H. Goldberg, L. W. Ripa, and J. Barenie, *J. Dental Res.,* **56**, 569 (1977).

21. G. Gallup, "Teens Name Favorite, Least Favorite Foods." (Press Release) (June 25, 1980).

22. D.H.E.W. *Ten-State Nutrition Survey, 1968–1970,* Vol. V. D.H.E.W. Publication No. (HSM) 72-8133.

23. D.H.E.W. "Dietary Intake of Persons 1–74 Years of Age in the United States." *Advancedata,* No. 6 (March 30, 1977).

24. R. M. Leverton, *J. Am. Dietetic Assoc.,* **53**, 13 (1968).

25. D. Sanjur, *The Professional Nutritionist,* **11**, 1 (1979).

26. J. A. Desor, L. S. Greens, and O. Maller, *Science,* **190**, 686 (1975).

27. G. Spagnoli, " 'Junk Foods' Rile Albany." *N.Y. Daily News* (March 30, 1977).

28. National Center for Health Statistics. *Monthly Vital Statistics Report—Health Examination Survey Data* (HRA) 76–1120, Vol. 25, No. 3, Supplement. (June 22, 1976).

29. Institute of Human Nutrition, "Nutrition and Exercise," *Nutrition and Health,* **2**(4), (1980).

30. Institute of Human Nutrition, "Nutrition and the Adolescent," *Nutrition and Health,* **2**(5), (1980).

31. L. Finberg, *Am. J. Dis. Childhood,* **130**, 362 (1976).

32. J. M. Axelson and D. S. Del Campo, *J. Nutrition,* **10**, 30 (1978).

PART 2

Nutrition under Conditions of Stress

5

Nutrition in the Pregnant Adolescent

PEDRO ROSSO, M.D. AND S. A. LEDERMAN, Ph.D.

Babies Hospital and Institute of Human Nutrition, Columbia University College of
Physicians and Surgeons, New York, New York

THE MAGNITUDE OF THE PROBLEM AND ITS DETERMINANTS

The rate of adolescent childbearing in the United States is the highest among the industrialized nations (1). As seen in Table 5-1 the rate of deliveries in the United States by women 19 years of age or younger is almost double that of England, nearly three times higher than in France or Sweden, and nearly 20 times higher than in Japan (2). Based on these rates, it has been estimated that approximately one million American adolescents become pregnant every year, or one of every ten girls between the ages of 15 and 19. Of this one million, approximately 600,000 give birth and approximately 25% of these give birth again within a year. The majority of these pregnancies and deliveries occur in girls who are 17 years old or older and only a small percentage are in the very young, 14 years old and under (2).

The relative importance of the various factors responsible for the high rate of adolescent pregnancy is not well established. In the last 35 years the age of puberty has been steadily decreasing and the average age at menarche in the United States is now 12.5 years, with approximately 13% of the population reaching puberty before age 11 (3). Obviously, this change has increased the proportion of sexually mature adolescents in the population and also has increased the length of time during which an adolescent may conceive before reaching adulthood.

Table 5-1.   Percentage of Births by Women 19 Years Old or Younger in Various Industrial Nations

Country	Percentage of All Births
United States	20
England	11
Sweden	7
France	7
Japan	1

[a]From L.M. Nix, (2).

Associated with these demographic and biological factors is a constellation of conditions that are part of the fabric of life in inner city populations of the United States where teenage pregnancy rates are highest. Nationally, the age-specific fertility rates, that is, the number of births per 1000 women of a specific age, are much higher in the black than in the white population (4). For any age group under 20 years of age, the fertility rate among blacks is more than two times the fertility rate of whites. When black–white fertility rates within a major city are compared, the difference becomes even more accentuated. For example, between 1950 and 1966 in the city of Baltimore, the fertility rates in black adolescents was four times higher than among white adolescents (4).

Surprisingly, the racial and socioeconomic aspects of adolescent pregnancies were not adequately analyzed in the early studies. As a result there is a considerable quantity of data in the literature that is very hard to interpret because of the many confounding variables not taken into consideration. Some of these early studies helped to foster ideas about teenage pregnancy which recent studies have shown to be erroneous, including the concepts that most women under 19 are "biologically immature" or that in the teenage mother there is a "competition between the needs for maternal growth and fetal growth."

OUTCOME OF PREGNANCY IN THE ADOLESCENT MOTHER

The outcome of pregnancy in adolescent mothers compares unfavorably with outcome in more mature women. The number of low birth weight babies (<2500 g) is considerably higher in mothers less than 19 years of age, while the percentage of infants weighing between 2500 and 3999 g at birth is lower than in more mature women (4). This difference suggests a downward shift in mean birth weight, a change that usually indicates unfavorable maternal conditions during gestation. Perinatal mortality is strongly associated with low birth weight. A higher incidence of low birth weight babies is always accompanied by higher death rates (4). Although neonatal mortality rates are higher in adolescent mothers, much of this difference disappears when racial composition is controlled. Nevertheless, neonatal mortality rates in both white and non-white infants are considerably higher in mothers under 15 than in older mothers (4) (Table 5-2).

Several studies have concluded that, in addition to delivering smaller infants with a higher risk of death in the neonatal period, teenage mothers have a higher incidence of premature delivery, cesarean sections due to cephalopelvic disproportion, toxemia, and anemia (5–8). However, there is some disagreement about the reasons for these findings. Basically, the question that has not been conclusively answered is whether the unfavorable outcome of pregnancy in the teenage mother is due solely to her own biological characteristics or to the environmental and social conditions to which she is exposed and which, ultimately, may influence the biological aspects. A recent analysis of data collected by the National Center for Health Statistics indicated that mothers under 18 years of age tend to have shorter gestations but the weight of the infant is appropriate for gestational age (9). This finding has been corroborated by a much smaller study carried out in Kansas City (10). This study suggested that when maternal factors such as low prepregnancy weight, low weight gain during pregnancy, smoking, the use of addicting drugs, or the use of alcoholic beverages are controlled, there are no differences

Table 5-2.   Neonatal Mortality of White and Nonwhite Infants by Age of Mother (Rate per 1000 Live Births)

	Neonatal Mortality		
Age of Mother	White	Nonwhite	Total
Under 15	32.1	46.5	41.2
15–19	20.4	30.9	22.7
20–24	15.9	25.3	17.3
25–29	15.3	24.2	16.6
30–34	17.0	26.4	18.3
Total	16.9	27.3	18.4

[a]From U.S. Dept. H.E.W. (4).

in mean birth weight, for a given gestational age, between adolescent mothers and mothers 20 to 34 years old. Only in very young mothers (under 14 years) is this issue unresolved, since too few subjects were included in this age group to draw valid conclusions. Other studies have also shown that some age-related negative effects on outcome disappear when the confounding variables are controlled (11–14).

The results of these studies strongly suggest that adolescent mothers share a disproportionate number of factors able to influence fetal growth negatively. However, when these factors are not present or are "controlled," the differences in pregnancy outcome between adolescent mothers and older mothers largely disappear. The situation is still unclear concerning the outcome in the very young mother since the importance of "gynecological age," or years since menarche, as an obstetric risk factor has not been adequately emphasized by most studies. As mentioned earlier, average age of menarche in the United States is 12.5 years. Hence studies of pregnant mothers under 15 years of age would include a high proportion of women with a gynecological age of less than 3 years. A carefully controlled study (15), in which mothers under 15 years of age were matched for various maternal and environmental variables with mothers over 20 years of age, found that the younger mothers had an increased incidence of toxemia and reduced pelvic inlet. However, the incidence of anemia, cesarean section, low birth weight, and perinatal mortality was similar. Although the rate of premature delivery was not statistically different in the two groups, the adolescent mothers showed a definite trend toward having shorter gestations. Nevertheless, even very young mothers do not seem to be at a marked biological disadvantage when compared with older mothers, except perhaps for the size of the pelvic inlet (Table 5-3).

NUTRITIONAL STATUS OF THE ADOLESCENT MOTHER

One of the environmental factors that can influence pregnancy outcome is maternal nutritional status. During the last decade several studies have investigated this important aspect (16–21). Unfortunately, it is difficult to ascertain the significance of these data since some of the studies are without an adequate control group, the number of the subjects is very small, gynecological age is not considered, and the information provided on the nutritional status of the subjects is inadequate. The largest and most detailed available study on the nutritional status of the adolescent

Table 5-3.   Pregnancy Performance of 471 Mothers Under 15 Years of Age and 19–25-year-old Matched Controls

	Percentages	
	Under 15	Controls
Anemia		
(Hb less than 10 g/dl)	5.6	6.0
Preeclampsia	34.2	25.3[b]
Pelvimetry		
(Inlet smaller than 85%)	7.4	2.8
Duration of pregnancy		
Less than 35 weeks	10.5	5.4
Less than 37 weeks	10.0	12.3
Cesarean sections	10.4	7.0
Infant weight		
1500–2499 g	15.0	12.5
Perinatal mortality	3.0	3.8

[a]From J. H. Duenholter, et al. (15).
[b]$p < 0.01$

mother included 550 pregnant teenagers, approximately 70% black and 30% white (16). Compared with the 1964 Recommended Dietary Allowances, the intake of the subjects was adequate in calories, protein, vitamin C, thiamine, and riboflavin. In contrast, calcium and iron intake was considered to be inadequate and vitamin A and niacin intake was lower than the norm but still within adequate limits. The biological assessment revealed the presence of iron deficiency anemia in 23% of the subjects and low vitamin A levels in a similar portion.

The levels of caloric and protein intake reported in this study are considerably higher than in other studies (18–20) and, unless a high percentage of the population was obese, they are not consistent with the reported finding that 46% of the subjects gained less than 25 lb during pregnancy.

In general, reported values of food intake in most of the available studies seem extremely low (average 1700 kcal/day) when compared with values found in older pregnant women (22, 23), and studies of pregnant adolescents consistently reveal inadequate intakes of calcium, iron, and vitamin A.

A recent study lends support to the concept that inadequate maternal nutrition may be responsible for the lower mean birth weight observed in teenage pregnancies. In this study (24), poor, pregnant girls attending a public school were divided into unsupplemented and supplemented groups. Important maternal characteristics were the same in the two groups. Nevertheless, the group that consumed the supplement (for a mean total intake of 8691 kcal and 529 g of protein as well as vitamins and minerals) had infants with a significantly higher mean birth weight than the infants of the unsupplemented group. A larger effect of supplementation was observed in girls below 16 years of age than in girls above that age, suggesting that nutritional status may be more marginal in the younger group.

THE NUTRITIONAL MANAGEMENT OF THE ADOLESCENT MOTHER

General Aspects

Considering the inadequacy of the available information, it seems difficult to derive guidelines for the most adequate nutritional management of a pregnant adolescent. In a rather empirical way, current recommendations are directed toward reaching two goals: (1) a dietary intake as close as possible to the RDAs and (2) a weight gain of at least 25 lb. This is basically the same type of dietary recommendation that is given to an older mother. This recommendation is probably adequate for most subjects but it is erroneous as an overall approach because it does not take into consideration individual characteristics and needs. This criticism also applies to the more mature woman; the major problem is that maternal nutritional status at the beginning of pregnancy varies considerably from one subject to the other. Some mothers are underweight, others are obese; some have iron deficiency, others have adequate iron stores. Obviously it is not appropriate to use the same dietetic recommendations for all pregnant women.

Several studies have shown that weight gain during pregnancy, especially in underweight women, has a positive influence on birth weight (25–27). Therefore, adequate weight gain should be the major consideration and guideline in planning and monitoring the dietetic counseling of a pregnant woman. There is evidence that in order to provide the fetus with adequate conditions for growth, the mother must reach a certain "critical" body weight which results in a 10% "excess" body weight over ideal body weight at delivery (28). Further maternal weight increments do not have a further positive influence on birth weight. However, an inadequate body weight gain has a negative influence on birth weight. It has been estimated that in order to reach that critical body weight, a woman with an adequate weight for height at the beginning of pregnancy needs to gain at least 25 to 30 lb during gestation. For a woman who had a deficit in weight for height at the beginning of pregnancy, 25 to 30 lb may not be enough. She must first make up for her initial deficit in body weight and on top of that, gain 25 to 30 lb. These recommendations, which are valid for mothers over 20 years of age, may not be strictly adequate for an adolescent mother. Theoretically, allowance should be made for growth, and therefore it is important to first establish the stage of development of the mother. The growth spurt of adolescence, as reflected by height increments, occurs as early as 10 years of age and as late as 14, with an average around 12.5 years of age (29). A similar variability occurs in weight "velocity." The average peak of weight gain occurs at 12.5 years of age, with some individuals reaching a peak velocity at 10.5 and others at 14.5 years of age (29). Menarche occurs when growth velocity is beginning to slow down, while other changes characteristic of sexual maturity, such as the development of the breasts and pubic hair, extend throughout the entire period of the growth spurt (29). Menarche, however, does not necessarily imply capacity to reproduce. It is generally agreed that early menstrual cycles tend to be irregular with a high incidence of anovular, and therefore infertile, cycles (30). Cases have been reported of pregnancy before the first menstruation or shortly thereafter but there seems to be little doubt that full fertility is not usually attained until some time, perhaps about 2 years, after menarche (31). At this time, the rate of growth has decelerated considerably but growth allowances should still be taken into consideration. A study has shown that for average girls, the 6-month weight increments decrease progressively following the age at which most of them had their menarche (12.5–13 years) (32). Two years later, when they are likely to be fully fertile, the 6-month weight increment is approximately 1 kg (2 lb). This weight increment must be computed in the recommendation of pregnancy weight gain (Table 5-4). For example, consider the hypothetical case of a 15-year-old with average body build who experienced menarche at 12.5 years. If at conception she weighed only 48 kg (105 lb) and was 167 cm tall, then according to available tables (33) she should be considered approximately 7 kg (15.4 lb) underweight. Her estimated growth increment for the next 9 months is 1.13 kg (2.58) lb). The average weight increment for pregnancy itself is 12.5 kg (27.5 lb). Hence this subject should gain approximately 20.6 kg (45.3 lb) for optimal fetal growth (Table 5-5). This seems a difficult undertaking, although the example used would be an extreme case. If the subject had had an adequate initial weight, 12.5

Table 5-4.   Six-monthly Weight Increments in a Representative Group of Girls (50th Percentile)[a]

	Body Weight Increments	
Age Intervals (years)	(kg)	(lb)
12.5–13	2.27	4.99
13–13.5	2.16	4.75
13.5–114	1.59	3.49
14 –14.5	1.31	2.88
14.5–15	1.08	2.37
15 –15.5	0.96	2.12
15.5–16	0.34	0.74
16 –16.5	0.68	1.49
16.5–17	0.45	0.99
17 –17.5	0.56	1.23
17.5–18	0.30	0.66

[a]From Roche *et al.* (32).

Table 5-5.   Weight Gain Recommendation for a 15-year-old Gravida

Basic data

Age	15 years
Age of menarche	12.5 years
Body weight at conception	48 kg (105.6 lb)
Body height at conception	62 cm (64 in.)
Adequate weight for height	55 kg (121 lb)

Recommendation

Estimated weight deficit	7 kg (15.4 lb)
Estimated growth increments (9 months)	1.13 kg (2.48 lb)
Average pregnancy gain	12.5 kg (27.5 lb)
Total weight to be gained	20.6 kg (45.3 lb)

kg (27 lb) would have been adequate to cover both her growth and pregnancy requirements. This appears to be an easier goal to reach. In support of these theoretical recommendations, one study (7) shows that a group of teenage mothers who gained more than 30 lb during gestation did not deliver infants weighing less than 2500 g.

Dietetic Recommendations

To be able to sustain adequate weight increments the pregnant teenager must receive adequate amounts of an appropriate diet which, in accordance with previous considerations, must be designed on an individual basis.

The *Recommended Dietary Allowances* (34) constitutes the most complete source of scientific information for establishing dietetic recommendations. This publication lists recommended nutrient intakes "designed for maintenance of good nutrition in practically all healthy people in the U.S.A." The recommended intakes are distinguished for three intervals during the teen years (11–14, 15–18, and 19–22) and are intended to allow for adolescent growth needs. A separate increment in intake is recommended for pregnancy. To determine the nutrient intake to be recommended for the pregnant adolescent, it is customary to use the age-appropriate recommendation and add to it the increment recommended for pregnancy. Table 5-6 shows the resulting recommendations for all the nutrients included in the RDAs. It must be pointed out that the value of RDAs for pregnant teens is clearly limited because pregnant teens are not merely adult gravidae who are still growing, as is implied by the adding of teen and pregnancy requirements. In addition, these recommendations are, to a large extent, guesses. The data for pregnancy are weak because they fail to account for changes occurring throughout gestation and because of the special difficulties of using radioisotope-labeled vitamins during pregnancy to establish requirements.

Similarly, there are few direct data on the needs of adolescents, as indicated in the text materials accompanying the RDA tabulations (34). Most of the adolescent recommendations are therefore derived by extrapolation or interpolation from other age groups with an allowance for the change in growth requirements. For the evaluation of the magnitude of maternal growth needs during pregnancy in teenagers, population averages are of little value, since pregnant teenagers as a group may include many more early maturers than the general teen population. For this reason, as previously discussed, it is worthwhile to assess gynecological age and growth potential as well as chronological age, prior to formulating a nutritional program for a specific teen.

It must also be considered that in many cases the nutrition prior to pregnancy was less than ideal. For example, the Ten-State Nutrition Survey (35), which emphasized low income populations, demonstrated that adolescents between 10 and 16 years of age had poorer nutritional status than any other age group. Nutrient deficits that may have developed before pregnancy must be compensated for, where possible, during pregnancy. Assessment of the individual's nutritional history and relevant laboratory and clinical findings are essential to an appropriate recommendation. Several nutrients deserve attention if the special circumstances surrounding teen pregnancies are considered.

Calories.   As indicated in Table 5-6, the recommended energy allowance for pregnant teens 14 years of age or less is 2700 kcal, a 200-kcal increment being allotted for maternal growth. Examination of height and weight velocity curves (36) reveals the large range of growth rates of, for example, 14-year-old girls. Late-maturing girls may be achieving their peak height velocity at this age, with height increments ranging from 2.5 to 3.7 cm/yr (3rd and 95th percentiles, respectively).

On the other hand, early maturers in all percentiles will have completed their height and weight increases by age 14. Since early maturers would be sexually active at an earlier age than late maturers, pregnant teenagers 14 years of age are more likely to have completed their growth than the average nonpregnant 14-year-old. Thus, their mean calorie requirement may not be as high as the average value for teen populations.

Table 5-6.   Food and Nutrition Board, National Academy of Sciences—Natio

	Age (years)	Weight (kg)	Weight (lb)	Height (cm)	Height (in.)	Pro-tein	Vita-min A (µg RE)	Vita-min D (µg)	Vita-min E (mg α−TE)	Vitamin C (mg)	Thia-mine (mg)
							Fat-Soluble Vitamins			_Water-So_	
Nonpregnant females	11−14	46	101	157	62	46	800	10	8	50	1.1
	15−18	55	120	163	64	46	800	10	8	60	1.1
	19−22	55	120	163	64	44	800	7.5	8	60	1.1
	23−50	55	120	163	64	44	800	5	8	60	1.0
Pregnant females	11−14					76	1000	15	10	70	1.5
	15−18					76	1000	15	10	80	1.5
	19−22					74	1000	12.5	10	80	1.5
	23−50					74	1000	10	10	80	1.4

ᵃDesigned for the maintenance of good nutrition of practically all healthy people in the U.

Recommending that fully grown pregnant teens consume fewer calories than those who are not fully grown has other nutritional ramifications. When calorie needs are reduced, there is less room for nutrient-poor, "empty calorie" food choices, which are frequently consumed by teens (16). Thus, although maternal growth may be a minor factor in determining the recommendations for most pregnant teens, altering spontaneous food choices may be more critical than in older gravidae. In addition, the percentage of low birth weight infants is higher among mothers under 15 years of age than in older women (4, 15, 37). As stated earlier, inadequate weight gain during pregnancy has been generally demonstrated to be associated with low birth weight (25, 26). Even in teens under 16 years old, a weight gain of more than 30 lb has been shown to prevent low birth weight (7).

It is particularly important to evaluate calorie needs and weight gain in pregnant teens in light of their current body weight. Pregnant teenagers are predominantly black and poor (37, 38). Both of these characteristics are associated with obesity in women (39). On the other hand, recent trends emphasizing the desirability of extreme leaness have resulted in an increase in the number of teenage girls below their ideal body weight. Both trends probably reflect the establishment of inappro-

arch Council Recommended Daily Dietary Allowances, Revised 1980[a]

uins				Minerals					
in NE)	Vitamin B₆ (mg)	Folacin (µg)	Vitamin B₁₂ (µg)	Calcium (mg)	Phosphorus (mg)	Magnesium (mg)	Iron (mg)	Zinc (mg)	Iodine (µg)
	1.8	400	3.0	1200	1200	300	18	15	150
	2.0	400	3.0	1200	1200	300	18	15	150
	2.0	400	3.0	800	800	300	18	15	150
	2.0	400	3.0	800	800	300	18	15	150
	2.4	800	4.0	1600	1600	450	*	20	175
	2.6	800	4.0	1600	1600	450	*	20	175
	2.6	800	4.0	1200	1200	450	*	20	175
	2.6	800	4.0	1200	1200	450	*	20	175

priate eating habits, which must be considered along with actual body weight when counseling pregnant teens. As previously discussed, it has been found that obese teens eat less (40) than nonobese teens and, in general, teen populations have a low intake of iron, calcium, and vitamins A and C (16, 41). Therefore, obese teens need to be specifically encouraged to achieve a normal, but not excessive, weight gain during pregnancy if optimal outcome is to be attained. Very lean girls must be advised that maintaining their low body weight would be detrimental and that a higher than average weight gain during gestation is desirable for them and their infants.

Protein.   Specific requirements for essential amino acids are not known for pregnancy. Nitrogen balance techniques have been the basis of most determinations of protein needs. Excessive or inadequate calorie intake can lower nitrogen balance and must be considered in evaluations of the adequacy of protein intake (34). The current allowances assume that protein utilization for growth is as efficient as utilization for mainte-nance in adults. Although this assumption has not been tested by experimentation, the increment allowed for growth is small (2 g/day) and may have little significance in diet evaluations.

An increase in protein intake of 30 g/day is currently recommended during pregnancy (34). This recommendation is based on limited data and is probably liberal. American diets tend to be high in protein, although among the poor, protein intake and quality may be low in specific individuals (39). Individual evaluation of dietary patterns of pregnant teens is desirable and should include consideration of the nature of the proteins consumed and the adequacy of calorie intake.

Iron.   In teens, as in adult women, iron status during pregnancy is particularly precarious. Several studies have shown that a large portion of teenage girls have low iron intake (16, 39) and low hemoglobin levels (35, 42, 43), although this is not a constant finding (37). Nevertheless, iron intake is generally low in teen populations (39) and anemia is a frequently cited nutritional problem of black females and of pregnant women generally. Irrespective of age, pregnant women are advised to take iron supplements during pregnancy to ensure adequate iron nutriture (34). Howver, many pregnant teens do not take prescribed supplements (44). This finding indicates that attention to dietary pat-terns that increase the intake of iron-rich foods may be especially important in teenage groups.

Calcium.   The recommended dietary allowance for calcium is 400 mg higher for pregnant women than for nonpregnant women (34). Teens that are still growing during gestation are advised to consume 1600 mg of calcium per day, double the amount for adult, nonpregnant women. This level of intake is difficult to achieve without hearty consumption of milk or milk products, yet milk consumption frequently stops and calcium intake has been found to be well below recommended levels in nonpregnant black women during the teen years (39). In addition, soda, which is high in phosphate content, may replace other beverages in the teen diet (16). Several studies suggest that a high ratio of dietary phosphate to calcium may seriously impair absorption of dietary calcium. Among black adolescents, lactase deficiency may further affect their willingness to increase milk consumption during gestation. Thus, even if the teen mother is fully grown, she is unlikely to have adequate calcium intake.

There is still, however, some question about the necessity for the high levels of calcium intake recommended in the RDAs, since adaptation to lower intakes are known to occur with time (34). Nevertheless, it would be wise to avoid requiring such adaptation during pregnancy. Hence any dietary changes that are recommended during pregnancy should be designed to ensure maintenance of adequate calcium intake, especially in those pregnant teens who are still growing. These changes may require some inventiveness if milk products will not be used.

Vitamin A.   Of all the fat-soluble vitamins, vitamin A intake has most often been found to be low in adolescent populations (16, 19). This finding is consistent with the observation that consumption of fresh fruits and vegetables is often poor among adolescents (39–41). With good counseling, it may be possible to increase the use of these nutritionally more desirable foods in place of the more generally used sweet, high-calorie snack items such as potato chips, ice cream, and candy.

Water-Soluble Vitamins.   Some studies suggest that there may be inadequate B-vitamin status in some teens. For example, low urinary riboflavin (16) and low intake of pantothenic acid (45), riboflavin (39), and folic acid (46) have been reported. Whether these findings all reflect true deficiencies or are partly the consequence of excessively high recommendations or inadequate knowledge of vitamin content of food for proper interpretation of the intake data is unclear. They do suggest, however, that special attention must be devoted to assessing vitamin status in pregnant teens, with appropriate laboratory tests where indicated. Unwillingness to consume milk, due to lactase deficiency, for example, may contribute to a risk of riboflavin deficiency.

Other Nutritional Factors. A thorough nutrition evaluation during gestation must include assessment of the role of alcohol, smoking, and consumption of other drugs. Consumption of these toxic materials has not been routinely explored in research on pregnant adolescents. Most studies do not evaluate the role of such factors in affecting outcome in the teen group. Nutritionists must make an effort to estimate the extent to which alcohol may replace other calories, or even be a primary hazard for the fetus of the teen mother, as it can be in older women. Young women, in particular, must be cautioned against smoking, drug taking, and caffeine consumption, since they are less likely than older women to be aware of the hazards to their child.

A review of the literature on nutrition in teen pregnancies shows that both from a theoretical and from a practical viewpoint, the available information is incomplete and outdated. Therefore, it is really not possible to make well founded and precise dietary recommendations. Many of the current standards may be unnecessarily high for nongrowing pregnant teens, but may be inadequate for the teen who is in the midst of the adolescent growth spurt or not in good mental and physical health. Existing guidelines can provide only a crude standard for individual dietary assessment.

It must also be recognized that it is difficult to achieve those nutritional changes which may prove desirable. Studies consistently show that many of the predominantly poor, black teens who make up the bulk of pregnant teenagers do not comply with dietary and medical advice, or present themselves too late in gestation for appropriate intervention (16). Outreach programs may have some salubrious effects, particularly where income constraints on food purchases may be reduced by encouraging participation in food stamp or WIC programs, but counseling difficulties remain substantial.

To some extent, these difficulties may be reduced if health professionals recognize that, contrary to earlier beliefs, social disabilities play a larger role in determining outcome in teen pregnancies than maternal growth does. This recognition focuses attention on more appropriate counseling techniques that treat the nutritional problems of pregnant teens in the local context of their social, psychological, and medical circumstances.

REFERENCES

1. W. H. Baldwin, Population Bulletin, Adolescent Pregnancy and Childbearing—Growing Concern for Americans, Washington, D.C., 29, 1976.
2. L. M. Nix, "Adolescent Pregnancy: Problems, Programs and New Directions," in Harel, S. Ed., *The at Risk Infant*, Excerpta Medica International Congress Series 492, Amsterdam–Oxford–Princeton, 1980, p. 19.
3. C. R. Cagas and H. D. Riley, *Am J. Dis. Child.*, **120**, 303 (1970).
4. "Relation of Nutrition to Pregnancy in Adolescence," in, *Maternal Nutrition and the Course of Pregnancy*, National Academy of Sciences, Washington, D.C., 1971, p. 139.
5. A. A. Marchetti and J. S. Menaker, *Am. J. Obstet. Gynecol.*, **59**, 1013 (1950).
6. F. C. Battaglia, T. M. Frazier, and A. E. Hellegers, *Pediatrics*, **32**, 902 (1963).
7. G. A. Webb, C. Briggs, and R. C. Brown, *Am. J. Obstet. Gynecol.*, **113**, 511 (1972).
8. D. G. Gill, R. Illsley, and L. H. Koplik, *Soc. Sci. Med.*, **3**, 549 (1970).
9. H. J. Hoffman, F. E. Lundin, L. S. Bakketeig, and E. E. Harley, "Classification of Birth by Weight and Gestational Age for Future Studies of Prematurity, in D. M. Reed and F. J. Stanley, *The Epidemiology of Prematurity*, Urban and Schwarzenberg, Baltimore–Munich, 1977, p. 297.
10. H. C. Miller and T. A. Merritt, *Fetal Growth in Humans*, Year Book Medical Pub., Chicago–London, 1979.
11. A. B. Elester and E. R. McAnarney, *Ped. Ann.*, **9**, 89 (1980).
12. R. P. Perkins, I. I. Nakashima, M. Mullin, L. S. Dubansky, and M. L. Chin, *Obstet. Gynecol.*, **52**, 179 (1978).
13. W. N. Spellacy, C. S. Mahan, and A. C. Cruz, *South. Med. J.*, **71**, 768 (1978).
14. F. L. Hutchins, N. Kendall, and J. Rubino, *Obstet. Gynecol.*, **54**, 1 (1979).
15. J. H. Duenhoelter, J. M. Jimenez, and G. Baumann, *Obstet. Gynecol.*, **46**, 49 (1975).
16. W. J. McGanity, H. M. Little, A. Fogelman, L. Jennings, E. Calhoun, and E. B. Dawson, *Am. J. Obstet. Gynecol.*, **103**, 773 (1969).
17. F. Smith, *Publ. Health Rep.*, **84**, 213 (1969).
18. H. J. Osofsky, P. T. Rizk, M. Fox, and J. Mondanaro, *J. Reprod. Med.*, **6**, 29 (1971).
19. J. C. King, S. H. Cohenout, D. H. Calloway, and H. N. Jacobson, *Am. J. Clin. Nutr.*, **25**, 916 (1972).
20. H. A. Kaminetzky, A. Langer, H. Baker, O. Frank, A. D. Thomson, E. D. Munves, A. Opper, F. C. Behrle, and B. Glista, *Am. J. Obstet. Gynecol.*, **115**, 639 (1973).
21. G. Ancri, E. H. Morse, and R. P. Clarke, *Am. J. Clin. Nutr.*, **30**, 568 (1977).
22. N. O. Lunell, B. Persson, and G. Sterky, *Acta Obstet. Gynecol. Scand.*, **48**, 187 (1969)
23. V. A. Beal, *J. Am. Diet. Assn.*, **58**, 312 (1971).
24. D. M. Paige, A. Cordano, E. D. Mellits, J. M. Baertl, and L. Davis, *J. Adol. Health Care* (in press).
25. N. J. Eastman, and E. Jackson, *Obstet. Gynecol.*, 23, 1002 (1968).
26. J. E. Singer, M. Westphal, and K. R. Niswander, *Obstet. Gynecol.*, **31**, 417 (1968).
27. K. R. Niswander, J. Singer, M. Westphal, and W. Weiss, *Obstet. Gynecol.*, **33**, 482 (1969)
28. P. Rosso, *Am. J. Clin. Nutr.* (in press).

29. W. A. Marshall, and J. M. Tanner, *Arch. Dis. Child.*, **44**, 291 (1969).

30. S. Matsumoto, M. Ozawa, Nogami and Ohashi, H.: *Gunma. J. Med. Sci.*, **12**, 119 (1963).

31. A. M. Thomson, "Pregnancy in Adolescence," in J. I. McKigney and H. N. Munro, Eds., *Nutrient Requirements in Adolescence*, MIT Press, Cambridge, 1976, p. 245.

32. A. F. Roche, "Aspects of Adolescent Growth and Maturation," in J. I. McKigney and H. N. Munro, Eds., *Nutrient Requirements in Adolescence*, MIT Press, Cambridge, 1976, p. 33.

33. D. B. Jelliffe, The Assessment of the Nutritional Status of the Community. WHO Monograph Series No. 53, 1966, p. 222.

34. National Research Council, Committee on Dietary Allowances, *Recommended Dietary Allowances*, 9th ed., National Academy of Sciences, Washington, D.C., 1980.

35. U.S. Department of Health, Education, and Welfare. Highlights, Ten-State Nutrition Survey, 1968–1970, Atlanta, Georgia.

36. J. M. H. Buckler, *A Reference Manual of Growth and Development*. Blackwell, Oxford–London–Edinburgh, 1979.

37. J. F. Hulka and J. T. Schaaf, *Obstet. Gynecol.*, **23**, 678 (1964).

38. T. A. Merritt, R. A. Lawrence, and R. L. Naeye, *Ped. Ann.*, **9**, 36 (1980).

39. S. Q. Haider, and M. Wheeler, *J. Am. Dietet. Assn.*, **77**, 677 (1980).

40. R. L. Huenemann, L. R. Shapiro, M. C. Hampton, and B. W. Mitchell, *J. Am. Dietet. Assn.*, **53**, 17 (1968).

41. Dietary habits of pregnant teenagers and their potential relation to pregnancy outcome. *Pub. Health Rep.*, **84**, 213 (1969).

42. I. R. Alton, *Persp. in Practice*, **74**, 667 (1979).

43. T. J. Muzzio, *Am. J. Obstet. Gynecol.*, **82**, 442 (1962).

44. E. S. Weigley, *J. Am. Dietet. Assn.*, **66**, 588 (1975).

45. S. H. Cohenour and D. H. Calloway, *Am. J. Clin. Nutr.*, **25**, 512 (1977).

46. W. A. Daniel, J. R. Mounger, and J. C. Perkins, *Am. J. Obstet. Gynecol.*, **111**, 233 (1971).

6

Nutrition and the Adolescent Athlete

NATHAN J. SMITH, M.D.

University of Washington School of Medicine, Seattle, Washington

More than six million high school students are currently participating in interscholastic sports programs and several million younger adolescents are involved in team sports at the junior high school level. Programs such as dance, swimming, and gymnastics are available to adolescents in most American communities. Along with the enormous increase in the numbers of both boys and girls participating in sports during the past decade there has been a marked increase in the number of different sports available to young people. A generation ago there were usually no interscholastic sports available to girls in most schools and only three or four organized for high school boys. Today over thirty different sports are approved for school competition for girls and a similar number are approved for high school boys. In various school systems, 20% to more than 60% of girls will be spending some of each day as young athletes. Boys with a variety of different interests and physical attributes can participate in one or more of the considerable variety of sports currently available. A high school boy is no longer limited in his choices of being only a football or basketball player if he is to have the benefit of high school athletics.

Sport participation can have a very positive influence on development during the years of adolescence. Security, self-esteem, peer and parent acceptance, and a host of desired personality traits can be strengthened. Obviously, an inappropriate or poorly directed sport experience can have a serious negative impact in all of these areas. The muscle work, exercise, and energy expenditure involved in regular athletic training contribute significantly to the vitality, well-being, and health of the adolescent. Regular energy expenditure is an essential contributor to a desired nutrient intake in the sedentary life-style imposed by the restrictive urban environment in which most adolescents live.

Young people have always sought opportunities to compare and compete with their newly acquired and changing physiques. In the past, young males have had the opportunity for such comparison and competition in the physically demanding work and chores that were part of daily living. Today opportunities for such comparison are available only on the fields and courts of sport. Girls have been no less concerned about comparing and competing in certain limited aspects of physical performance and in various domestic and social skills. During the past decade young women have come to experience the vitality, fitness, and enjoyment from regular exercise and have prompted the creation of many new opportunities for sport participation.

The new expanding population of adolescent athletes recognizes food as the source of energy for competition and training as well as a major determinant of body composition; the degree of fatness or leanness, the level of hydration, and so on. Diet practices and food are known to be important factors influencing success or failure in sports. Athletic participation has created in this large segment of the adolescent population intense concern with food intake and nutrition-related fitness.

THE ATHLETE'S DAILY DIET

The energy used in the training for all active energy-expending sports, such as swimming, basketball, soccer, tennis, is supplied in large part through the aerobic and anaerobic metabolism of tissue stores of carbohydrate available as muscle and liver glycogen (1). The athlete should know that the body's capacity to store this important source of energy is distinctly limited. Tissue glycogen stores will be optimally available to meet the energy demands of training and competition only if replenished by regular, periodic food intakes. Regular energy intakes are most dependably experienced in a diet pattern of regular mealtime eating. The common practice of one large eating experience during much of the evening and only unpredictable and irregular snacking during the day is a compromising schedule of energy intake for an athlete participating in late afternoon practice sessions. Tissue glycogen stores are normally limited to 1000 to 1500 kcal and when these are replenished only late in the evening, they will be essentially exhausted by midafternoon if there has not been a meaningful intake of energy during the intervening daytime hours.

Food energy must be taken both at regular intervals and in sufficient amount to maintain a desired competing weight during the several weeks or months of competing season. The adequacy of total energy intake is monitored by regularly recording body weight. Scheduled weighing is essential in monitoring the nutritional status of the serious young athlete. Involuntary weight loss reflects negative energy balance; that is, more energy is being expended than is being taken in. This is the most common nutrition-related problem encountered among young athletes. Overcommitment to a host of academic and social interests in addition to commitments to training may leave "no time for eating." The energy requirements of a rapidly growing adolescent boy expending large amounts of energy in an active sport program may be greater than can be met by the limited food available in a poverty home. Monitoring weight is essential in assuring the adequacy of energy intake.

Athletes should know that even the most rigorous and demanding training efforts do not increase the body's needs for any specific nutrient (2). A mixed diet adequate in amount to satisfy the energy demands of training will provide an abundance of all essential nutrients. The athlete with this knowledge will confidently accept that vitamin, mineral, or protein supplements are useless, needlessly expensive, and potentially dangerous. It is often helpful for concerned young people to record their total dietary intake for a few days, and evaluate their food selections using some simple reference such as the "four food groups." Documenting an appropriately varied food selection, the athletes can be reassured that their diet satisfies the need for all essential nutrients. The only nutrition supplement appropriate for young athletes is an iron supplement that may be required for some 10 to 20% of menstruating women in the United States (3). Women and young girls in sports programs will have a similar need for an iron supplement.

ALTERING BODY COMPOSITION: ACHIEVING COMPETING WEIGHT

The majority of adolescents in sports programs seriously strive to optimize their athletic performance. In recent years coaches and athletes have come to identify specific levels of body fatness that are associated with elite performance in many sports (4) (Table 6-1).

Excess body fat is known to reduce speed and quickness, limit endurance, and contribute nothing to strength. Reducing body fat to a

Table 6-1.   Relative Body Fat Values for Males and Females in Various Sports[a]

Sport	Males Fat %	Females Fat %
Baseball/softball	12–14	16–26
Basketball	7–10	16–27
Football	8–18	—
Gymnastics	4–6	9–15
Ice hockey	13–15	—
Jockeys	12–15	—
Skiing	7–14	18–20
Soccer	9–12	—
Speed skating	10–12	—
Swimming	5–10	14–26
Track and field		
Sprinters	6–9	8–20
Middle distance runners	6–12	8–16
Distance runners	4–8	6–12
Discus	14–18	16–24
Shot put	14–18	20–30
Jumpers and hurdlers	6–9	8–16
Tennis	14–16	18–22
Volleyball	8–14	16–26
Weightlifting	8–16	—
Wrestling	4–12	—

[a]The values represent the range of means reported in various published and unpublished studies.

minimum compatible with a high degree of fitness and health is highly desirable for athletes competing in a variety of sports such as distance running, gymnastics, figure skating, and particularly in those sports where the athletes are matched on the basis of weight (wrestling, lightweight rowing, weight lifting, etc.). A goal for athletes in all of these sports is to have the maximum strength, endurance, and quickness for every unit of body weight taken into the contest.

An athlete who wants to reduce body fatness to a level desired for competition will need a well-planned program of energy-expending exercise and a prescribed diet that will be sufficient to support the needs of training while protecting muscle tissue from being used as a source of energy (5). The amount of fat to be lost is estimated by assessing existing level of body fat and projecting the optimal level of fatness desired for the specific sport. These assessments are made using either a skin fat fold caliper or hydrostatic weighing. For the average adolescent boy or girl athlete a desired rate of fat reduction in achieving a fit fatness level is approximately 2 lb/week. This fat reduction will be accomplished by creating a negative energy balance of approximately 1000 kcal/day. Energy expenditure is increased in training activities so that the desired negative energy balance will occur while the athlete has a food energy intake of no less than 2000 kcal/day. This restricted caloric intake is maintained for the few weeks that are required to reduce fatness to the desired level. Once the desired level of fatness has been achieved, caloric intake is increased to maintain a desired competing weight and satisfy the energy needs of athletic training and normal growth. Weight and the level of fatness should be monitored and remain stable during the competing season.

The increasing concern for reduced levels of fatness to optimize competing potential in sports and the large number of young people making a serious commitment to competing has generated a nutrition-related problem that is being encountered with increasing frequency (6). Each season we are seeing athletes who are suffering from precipitous weight loss, having developed a striking aversion to food as they become overzealous in reducing body fat. When food must be eaten there may be self-induced vomiting, referred to by athletes as "flipping." The consequences of this aversion and often total avoidance of food are similar to the findings in any patient with starvation, such as that seen in anorexia nervosa. There is rapid loss of body fat, some muscle wasting, and in girls, amenorrhea.

The food aversion and precipitous weight loss in the athlete differs in several aspects from typical anorexia nervosa. Males are more frequently involved than females, because of the larger population of males seriously involved in athletic training. The weight loss occurs more precipitously as high energy-expending training schedules are maintained while there may be essentially no intake of food. Because of close association with coaches and teammates the athlete who has developed an aversion to food is usually recognized relatively early when there is an unavoidable deterioration of athletic performance. Individuals with this problem are high performing athletes, unusually talented students, and high achievers with an all consuming fear of failure to achieve what may be unattainable goals in sports, or in some social or academic activity. The early recognition, the presence of supporting teammates with a sincere interest in the person's well-being, and the strengths and talents of the individual himself, all contribute to a favorable prognosis for reversing the avoidance of food and establishing a desired food intake. Sincere and sympathetic counseling on a daily and follow-up basis by the family doctor or team physician is usually effective. Psychiatric consultation is rarely needed.

MEETING THE ENERGY DEMANDS OF SPECIFIC SPORTS

The energy needs of different sports are satisfied by different energy mechanisms (7). Short-term events, such as the sprints and gymnastic events, as well as field events such as the pole vault and long jump, all have their energy needs supplied by ATP and phosphocreatine stored in small amounts in muscle tissue. Maintaining a regular intake of fluids and small, high carbohydrate meals during what are often two or more days of competition satisfies the nutrition and energy needs of these events.

Planning for the regular intake of fluids and appropriate food becomes of increased importance in preparing for contests of longer duration that require more intense energy expenditure. The running games (basketball, tennis, soccer, etc.) and sports such as rowing and wrestling all demand intense expenditure of both aerobically and anaerobically generated energy over a significant time period. Teams and individual athletes involved in these sports are advised to have a well-planned diet for 3 or 4 days prior to serious competition. The diet should be high in carbohydrate, low in residue, and avoid excessive salt intake. When a tournament or series of games extends over a period of 2, 3, or more days a precise plan of what, where, and when the athletes will eat can be of great advantage. Well-planned meals provide an ideal time to make readjustments in team morale and give the athletes confidence that their food and energy needs are being optimally provided for.

Energy metabolism is efficient only in the presence of a good state of hydration. The fluid needs and replacement of the sweating athlete are best satisfied with water. Clean, cool water provided in generous amounts in sanitary containers is the ideal beverage for the athlete. The state of hydration during several hours or days of competition is effectively monitored by frequent nude weighing. Water intakes should be sufficient to maintain an initial precompeting weight. The various electrolytes and minerals lost in sweat are amply replaced with a varied diet sufficient in amount to meet the energy needs of the active athlete.

It is helpful to inform the athlete that sweat is a very hypotonic solution, particularly in the well-conditioned athlete acclimatized to vigorous exercise in a warm environment. The sweating athlete is losing much more water than salt relative to other isotonic body fluids. Concentrated or even isotonic beverages and salt tablets can only contribute to hypernatremic dehydration. The widely promoted "athlete drinks" containing varying amounts of glucose and electrolytes eliminate the sensation of thirst by creating sensations of satiety that discourage much needed fluid intakes. The electrolytes in these drinks satisfy no specific need of the well-nourished athlete. Probably nowhere but in the intense environment of competitive sport would otherwise rational individuals propose quenching the thirst of sweating athletes with salt water.

Scandinavian exercise physiologists demonstrated with serial muscle biopsy studies that duration of exercise performance was influenced by the concentration of glycogen in specific muscle fibers (1). High concentrations of muscle glycogen prolonged the period of exercise in laboratory study and improved athletic performance in endurance-type contests. Clinical observation suggests that performance may improve in nonendurance-type contests that demand an intense expenditure of both aerobic and anaerobic energy over shorter periods.

Glycogen concentration in muscle is maximized by 3 to 4 days of intense training of the specific muscle groups to be involved in competition while receiving a diet of very restricted carbohydrate content. This period of training and restricted carbohydrate intake is followed by 3 or 4 days of sharply reduced training activity while taking a diet that provides 1000 to 1500 kcal of residue-free carbohydrate. This carbohydrate source may be conveniently and predictably provided by sweetened beverages, hard candies, or a caloric supplement product commonly used in hospitals, polycose (R). This 8-day diet and training plan maximizes the glycogen content of the specific muscle fibers to be used in an important competition. In addition, it provides the athlete with a well-defined training and diet schedule for the week before an important event. This program is suitable only for the preparation for two or three important competitions during a competing season, is in no way proposed as a routine training diet, and should be tried by the serious athlete on a pilot, experimental basis early in the season to validate its acceptability and benefit for the individual.

IRON DEFICIENCY AND ATHLETIC PERFORMANCE

As reported elsewhere in this volume, iron deficiency is encountered with varying frequency in certain sex, age, and socioeconomic groups in the United States. Adolescent girls in all economic groups and adolescent males, particularly from low income families, are known to be at risk for iron deficiency. Those adolescents lacking in iron to a degree that they develop frank iron deficiency anemia do not commonly enter sports programs, or they drop out quite promptly. However, 8 to 10 % of girls "trying out" for scholastic sports programs may be found to be suffering from tissue-iron depletion identified with low levels of plasma ferritin and transferrin saturation. These individuals will usually have hemoglobin concentrations well within the range of normal. Finch and his associates have reproduced an animal model in the rat of tissue-iron depletion without anemia (7). The tissue-iron depleted nonanemic animals have been found to have compromised exercise performance. Aerobic energy metabolism has been shown to be altered, with the exercising rats utilizing anaerobic energy sources to an abnormal degree. The limited exercise tolerance is associated with abnormally high post-exercise concentrations of blood lactate. Clinical observation of varsity women athletes suggested that there was a similar limitation of exercise performance in those found to be iron depleted. Currently, iron-depleted women athletes are being shown under laboratory control to have limited exercise tolerance, high postexercise blood lactate levels, and striking responses in these measures after 10 days of iron therapy.

Large numbers of Americans are currently experiencing the benefits of enjoyable, regular exercise. Adolescents, both boys and girls, are pursuing more active life-styles and many are active participants in sports programs. Benefits in both physical well-being and in strengthening several aspects of developing behavior are coming from their increased sport participation. Sincere interest in athletic endeavors often provides the adolescents, known to be a nutritional risk, an effective motivation to upgrade their nutritional status through more desirable dietary practices.

REFERENCES

1. E. Hultman, in J. Parizkova and V. A. Rogozkin, Eds., *Nutrition, Physical Fitness and Health*, University Press, Baltimore, 1978.
2. J. Mayer and B. Bullen, *Physiol. Rev.*, **40**, 369 (1960).
3. J. D. Cook, C. A. Finch, and N. J. Smith, *Blood*, **48**, 449 (1976).
4. J. H. Wilmore, in N. J. Smith, Ed., *Sports Medicine for Children and Youth*, Ross Laboratories, Columbus, Ohio, 1979, p. 68.
5. N. J. Smith, *Food for Sport*, Bull Publishing, Palo Alto, 1976.
6. N. J. Smith, *Pediatrics*, **66**, 139 (1980).
7. C. A. Finch, L. R. Miller, A. R. Inamdar, R. Person, K. Seiler, and B. Mackler, *J. Clin. Invest.*, **58**, 447 (1976).

PART 3

Specific Nutrient Deficiencies

7

Iron Deficiency in Adolescents

PHILIP LANZKOWSKY, M.D., F.R.C.P., D.C.H.

State University of New York at Stony Brook and Long Island Jewish–Hillside Medical Center, New Hyde Park, New York

Iron deficiency is the most common nutritional deficiency and is widespread throughout the world. It is especially prevalent in infancy, in adolescence, and during pregnancy. The limited concentration of iron in many diets, the need for iron for growth, and the limited human ability to absorb dietary iron, as well as the high prevalence of parasitism and gastrointestinal blood loss in some populations, make infants, children, and adolescents vulnerable to negative iron balance and iron-deficiency anemia.

IRON ABSORPTION

Iron can probably be absorbed from any part of the gastrointestinal tract, although absorption is greatest in the duodenum and diminishes progressively in the more distal portion of the bowel.

The mucosal cell has two important roles in iron absorption: (1) mucosal uptake and (2) transfer of iron from the mucosal cell to the lamina propria, where it enters the plasma (1, 2). Both steps represent energy-dependent, active transport processes.

The quantity of iron absorbed after digestion is influenced by the following intraluminal and extraluminal factors:

Intraluminal factors:
  Amount of iron
  Type of iron
Relation to food:
  Presence or absence of food
  Nature of food
  Enhancing substances
  Inhibiting substances
Role of gastrointestinal tract:
  Gastric factors
  Pancreatic factors
  Bile
Extraluminal factors:
  Body iron stores
  Erythropoietic activity
  Growth

Intraluminal Factors

Amount of iron.   Increasing the amount of iron ingested increases the amount absorbed, even though the percentage of absorption is smaller with larger amounts of iron (3).

Type of Iron.   Ferrous iron is absorbed better than ferric iron. Heme iron, accounting for 80% of the soluble iron compounds in meat, is absorbed in a highly efficient manner and has a high nutritive value in meeting the body's needs for iron. The absorption of heme iron occurs by a mechanism different from that involved in the absorption of nonheme iron present in food or inorganic iron (4) and is not altered by the status of iron stores and iron demand, the presence of ascorbic acid, phytates, or chelating agents.

Relation to Food

Presence or Absence of Food.   Absorption of iron is reduced by approximately 50% by merely mixing ferrous salts in food.

Nature of Food.   Food iron ultimately must be converted to the ferrous form to be absorbed (5). Since the ease with which this conversion is accomplished differs according to the nature of the iron compound, the availability of food iron is quite variable. The range of iron absorption from biosynthetically labeled food is 1 to 22%. Meat and animal products are at the upper end and foods of vegetable origin at the lower end of this range. Fish muscle and animal muscle have an enhancing effect on the absorption of iron from vegetable foods, whereas milk, butter, and eggs are animal protein foods which do not enhance the absorption of vegetable iron. Iron present in vegetable or plant sources is absorbed less well than iron in animal tissues (a large portion of which is heme iron). If animal and plant sources of food iron are fed in combination, the absorption of iron from the vegetable sources is increased significantly. The reason for this may be that several of the amino acids, particularly cystine, lysine, and histidine, have been found to be effective in increasing the absorption of ferric iron. When amino acids are added to a vegetable diet, an increase in the absorption of vegetable iron is demonstrated when the amino acids are present in a proportion similar to that found in fish muscle. In foods derived from grains, iron often forms a stable complex of phytates, and only small amounts of such iron can be converted to the absorbable form (6). Similarly, the iron in egg yolk is not readily absorbed, probably because it is complexed with phosphates or phosphoproteins. The exact nature of iron in many other foods is not known. However, it appears to be mainly in the ferric state, much of it as ferric hydroxide or loosely bound to organic molecules such as sugars, citrates, lactate, and the amino acids.

Enhancing Substances.   These include ascorbic acid and other reducing substances, amino acids, and simple sugars, such as lactose and fructose, to a greater degree than sucrose or glucose. Chelation with these substances greatly enhances the subsequent absorption of iron, since the chelation in the acid medium of the stomach may maintain inorganic iron in a more soluble and readily absorbable form within the small bowel lumen.

Inhibiting Substances.   Compounds forming insoluble complexes with iron, such as phosphate, phytates (phosphorus-containing salts of phytic acid), and oxalates, decrease absorption.

Role of Gastrointestinal Tract

Gastric Factors. The acid gastric juice is a medium in which solubilization and reduction of iron are favored; consequently, absorption of ferric iron is impaired in subjects with gastrectomy or achlorhydria (7). The gastric juice of healthy people contains a high-molecular-weight iron-binding protein designated *gastroferrin* (8). Normally there is sufficient gastric juice to bind the 15 mg of iron present in a typical day's diet. This binding substance is not firm and iron is rapidly removed from the gastric factor by EDTA and transferrin. The iron-binding protein provides a mechanism, along with other natural ligands, in the chelation of soluble iron in the acid milieu of the stomach, maintaining solubility in the alkaline medium of the duodenum, the site of iron absorption.

Although some results support the concept that gastroferrin production is concerned with the regulation of iron absorption in health, these observations have been seriously contested. No differences have been found in the iron-binding content of the gastric juice between patients with hemochromatosis and controls (9) and some workers have found higher levels in iron-deficient subjects than in controls.

Pancreatic Factors. Pancreatic secretions have been implicated in iron absorption. Pancreatic enzymes may split iron-protein complexes and make iron available for absorption. Bicarbonate secreted by the pancreas, on the other hand, raises pH and induces formation of poorly absorbed iron complexes. Well-controlled studies with pancreatic insufficiency, however, have failed to show either iron excess or increased absorption of iron. Additionally, more recent studies indicate that the effect of pancreatic extract on iron absorption is nonspecific.

Bile. Bile facilitates iron absorption (10). Exclusion of bile from the intestine decreases absorption of food iron and iron salts. Bile contains ascorbic acid, which forms soluble chelates with iron, thus possibly enhancing iron absorption.

Extraluminal Factors

Iron Stores. The presence of iron deficiency, even at a time when depleted iron stores are not accompanied by changes in serum iron, hemoglobin levels, or iron-turnover rates, increases iron absorption. Thus the highest levels of absorption of dietary iron occur during periods of most rapid growth. Increased iron stores are associated with decreased iron absorption. Normal subjects absorb 5 to 10% of dietary iron, compared with about 20% in iron-deficient patients.

Erythropoietic Activity.   Increased erythropoietic activity in the marrow even if iron stores are already adequate (e.g., hemorrhage, hemolysis, ascent to a high altitude) increases iron absorption, and diminished erythropoiesis decreases iron absorption.

Growth.   Investigators have observed high rates of absorption of iron in early infancy which decrease rapidly with age to the level observed in adults. It has been demonstrated that growth is associated with increased demand for iron regardless of hemoglobin level. The percentage of iron absorption, independent of age, is linearly related to weight gain.

PREVALENCE OF IRON DEFICIENCY

Although the incidence of iron-deficiency anemia is high in infancy, it also exists in schoolchildren and during preadolescence. An incidence of iron deficiency of 5.5% in inner-city schoolchildren ranging in age from 5 to 8 years has been demonstrated, as well as an incidence of 2.6% in preadolescent children and 25% in pregnant teenage girls (11).

It has been observed by many investigators that there is a higher prevalence of iron-deficiency anemia in black than in white children. This was also apparent in a survey conducted by the author (Table 7-1) (12). Although no socioeconomic group is spared, the incidence of iron-deficiency anemia in large population groups is inversely proportional to economic status. The apparent role of ethnic and socioeconomic factors in the prevalence of iron-deficiency anemia is probably related to dietary habits, since foods of high iron content are probably less available to low-income groups. However, iron deficiency among adolescents has been found at all levels of economic status, in both sexes, and in all races (13).

Tables 7-2 and 7-3 show the mean and various percentiles for hemoglobin and transferrin saturation levels in adolescents 12–17 years of age in a national child health survey.

Table 7-1.   Hemoglobin Levels in Children of Different Ethnic Groups Aged 6 to 36 Months Attending Well-Baby Clinics[a]

	Black	Hispanic	White
Number	177	158	82
Mean hemoglobin, g/dl	10.9	11.4	12.1
Percent < 10.0 g/dl	21.0	11.0	2.0

[a]Significant differences ($p < 0.001$) among ethnic groups.

Table 7-2.   Hemoglobin Levels 12–17 Years of Age (National Child Health Survey—CDC)

		Mean ± 1 SD	5th Percentile	50th Percentile	95th Percentile
Males	White	14.3 ± 1.1	12.5	14.3	16.0
	Black	13.5 ± 1.3	11.6	13.4	15.5
Females	White	13.3 ± 0.9	11.9	13.4	14.9
	Black	12.4 ± 1.0	11.0	12.5	13.8

Table 7-3.   Transferrin Saturation Levels 12–17 Years of Age (National Child Health Survey—CDC)

		Mean ± 1 SD	10th Percentile	50th Percentile
Males	White	26.6 ± 9.1	16.1	25.4
	Black	26.1 ± 9.1	16.8	23.7
Females	White	26.1 ± 9.8	14.1	24.7
	Black	24.1 ± 9.5	12.1	23.4

ETIOLOGIC FACTORS IN IRON DEFICIENCY

The most common factors that contribute to the development of iron deficiency are insufficient dietary intake of iron, rapid growth, and blood loss. Many cases result from a combination of all three.

Dietary Factors

One of the major factors in the pathogenesis of iron-deficiency anemia is inadequate iron intake. Tables 7-4 and 7-5 show normal daily iron requirements calculated according to age and condition of various groups.

In adolescence, because of the growth spurt and (for girls) menstrual loss, there is an increase in iron requirements. A menstruating adolescent requires 1.6 to 1.85 mg of iron each day as replacement or 16 to 18.5 mg daily of dietary iron. Nonmenstruating adolescents require only 1.25 mg/day as replacement or about 12.5 mg daily of dietary iron (5 to 10% absorption). In some teenage boys and in many menstruating girls, a negative iron balance develops, with loss of iron stores, despite average nutrition. Iron balance in adolescence is shown in Table 7-6.

Table 7-4. Normal Daily Iron Requirements (mg)

	Normal Loss	Menses	Pregnancy	Growth	Total Requirement
Infants Aged 1 Year	0.25	—	—	0.8	1.05
Children Aged 7 Years	0.5	—	—	0.3	0.8
Pubertal Females	0.75	0.6	—	0.5	1.85
Menstruating Females	1.0	0.6	—	—	1.6
Pregnant Females	1.0	—	1.5	—	2.5
Adolescent Males	0.75	—	—	0.5	1.25

Table 7-5. Daily Dietary Iron Requirements in Adolescents

	Boys—Years of Age			Girls—Years of Age		
	9–12	12–15	15–18	9–12	12–15	15–18
Department of Health, U.K. 1969	13	14	15	13	14	15
World Health Organization 1974	5–10	9–18	5–9	5–10	12–24	14–28
National Research Council 1974	18	18	18	18	18	18

Table 7-6. Iron Balance in Adolescents

Iron intake (average):
Food iron	10–12 mg/dl
Absorption	10% or less
Iron absorbed	1.0–1.2 mg/day

Iron losses:	Male	Female
Exfoliation, body fluids, mg/day	0.75	0.75
Menstrual loss, mg/dl		0.6
Total losses	0.75	1.35
Growth needs, mg/dl	0.5	0.5
Total average iron requirement	1.25	1.85

In teenage pregnancies, additional iron (about 400 to 1000 mg) is required to satisfy fetal demand, increased maternal red blood cell volume, and blood loss at delivery. Lactation adds 0.5 to 1.0 mg/day to iron losses. Since iron stores are less than 350 mg in at least two-thirds of young women, significant maternal anemia may develop if supplemental iron is not provided during this period.

Table 7-7 lists the iron content of typical foods.

Table 7-7. Iron Contents of Foods

Food	Iron (mg)	Unit
Milk	0.5–1.5	liter
Eggs	1.2	each
Cereal, fortified	3.0–5.0	ounce
Vegetables		
Yellow	0.1–0.3	ounce
Green	0.3–0.4	ounce
Meats		
Beef, lamb, beef liver	0.4–2.0	ounce
Pork, liver, bacon	6.6	ounce
Fruits	0.2–0.4	ounce

Growth Factors

At puberty the weight doubles over a period of 7 years, with a gain of about 30 kg in weight for boys and a little less for girls. This rate requires 1200 mg of iron, or 170 mg/year, or 0.5 mg/day. This estimate is for growth alone; in girls an additional 0.6 mg/day is needed to compensate for menstrual loss.

Table 7-8 shows hemoglobin and blood volume changes in adolescence and Table 7-9 shows the iron requirements for 50th percentile adolescents indicating that lean body mass is very important in determining iron requirements. Body composition is more important in determining iron requirements than weight (14).

Blood Loss

Table 7-10 lists sources of blood loss leading to iron deficiency while Table 7-11 summarizes the factors affecting iron need in adolescence.

CLINICAL MANIFESTATIONS OF IRON-DEFICIENCY ANEMIA

It is well established that iron deficiency is a systemic disorder involving multiple systems rather than a purely hematologic condition associated with anemia. The early phases of iron-deficiency anemia are not associated with clearly recognizable signs or symptoms, and its develop-

Table 7-8.   Hemoglobin and Blood Volume Changes in Adolescence[a]

Age	12 Years		16 Years	
	Boys	Girls	Boys	Girls
Hemoglobin (gm/dl	13.2	12.2	15.4	14.0
Blood volume (ml)	2500	2500	6000	3500

[a]Hemoglobin concentration increases 0.5 to 1.0 gm/dl/yr (0.5 g/dl in 55-kg boy = 50 mg Fe).

Table 7-9.   Iron Requirements for 50th Percentile Adolescents[a]

Boys	42 mg iron/kg
Girls	31 mg iron/kg

[a]Reason: In preadolescence lean body mass (LBM) is the same for boys and girls. At the end of adolescence, LBM in boys is 2 times that of girls. So body composition not weight is more important.

Table 7-10.   Sources of Blood Loss

Gut

  Primary iron-deficiency anemia resulting in gut alteration with blood loss aggravating existing iron deficiency

  Hypersensitivity to whole cow's milk ? due to heat-labile protein, resulting in blood loss and exudative enteropathy

  Anatomic gut lesions, e.g., varices, hiatus hernia, ulcer, leiomyomata, ileitis, Meckel's diverticulum, duplication of gut, hereditary telangiectasia, polyps, colitis, hemorrhoids; exudative enteropathy due to underlying bowel disease, e.g., allergic gastroenteropathy, intestinal lymphangiectasia.

  Gastritis due to aspirin ingestion, adrenocortical steroids, indomethacin, phenylbutazone.

  Intestinal parasites, e.g., hookworm (Necator americanus)

  Henoch-Schönlein purpura

Gallbladder: hemocholecyst

Lung: pulmonary hemosiderosis, Goodpasture's syndrome, defective iron mobilization with IgA deficiency

Nose: recurrent epistaxis

Uterus: Menstrual loss

Heart: Intracardiac myxomata, valvular prostheses or patches

Kidney: Traumatic hemolytic anemia, hematuria, nephrotic syndrome (urinary loss of transferrin), hemosiderinurias (chronic intravascular hemolysis, e.g., paroxysmal noctural hemoglobinuria, paroxysmal cold hemoglobinuria, March hemoglobinuria)

Extracorporeal: hemodialysis, trauma

ment is slow and insidious. Pallor, irritability, anorexia, and listlessness usually direct attention to the disorder. These symptoms are noticed only when there has been a significant fall in the hemoglobin level.

Except for pallor of the skin and mucous membranes and occasionally a slightly enlarged spleen, the patient presents no significant physical abnormalities. In patients with severe anemia a soft, blowing, apical

Table 7-11.   Factors Affecting Fe Need in Adolescence

Needs
  Hemoglobin concentration increases 0.5 – 1.0 gm/dl/year (0.5 gm = 50 mg Fe)
  Velocity of growth. Growing at 97th percentile doubles Fe requirements
    compared to growth at 3rd percentile. Peak weight gain: boys 10 kg/year
    (300 mg Fe); girls 9 kg/year (280 mg Fe)
  Body composition: (Lean body mass) > in boys
                     (Blood volume) girls 3500 ml; boys 6000 ml
  Pregnancy
    Basal losses 220 mg
    Increase maternal red cell mass 500 mg
    Fetal requirements 290 mg
    Placental requirement 25 mg

Loss:
  Skin, bowel, urine
  Menstrual 30 ml/period (175 mg Fe/yr).

Amount and availability:
  Recommended daily dietary allowance in U.S.A.: 18 mg
  Because of variability of growth spurt (onset, rate, cessation) 18 mg Fe/day
    should be provided from 10 – 18 years

systolic murmur is frequently heard. Koilonychia (concave nails) has
been observed in severe, long-standing iron-deficiency anemia.

Iron deficiency affects many organ systems in the body, apart from
the hemopoietic system.

Gastrointestinal Tract

Anorexia is a common and early symptom of iron-deficiency anemia and
correction of iron deficiency results in improved appetite. Among
children with iron-deficiency anemia there is a marked preponderance
of underweight children; when iron is given to them, accelerated weight
gains occurs and produces a normal distribution curve (15).

Pica, derived from the Latin word meaning magpie, is a perversion of
appetite with persistent and purposeful ingestion of apparently unsuit-
able substances, seemingly of no nutrient value. Pica has been considered a symptom of iron-deficiency anemia, even though a number of

etiologic factors—nutritional, psychologic, socioeconomic, cultural, and organic—have been implicated in it. Pica has been shown by the author to be related to iron-deficiency anemia (16), and this has been confirmed by others. A group of children with pica, all of whom had iron deficiency, were all cured of their pica and iron-deficiency anemia by the administration of iron. A double-blind trial of the value of iron in the treatment of pica has revealed that pica associated with iron-deficiency anemia can be cured by iron.

Atrophic glossitis, dysphagia, esophageal webs usually at the cricopharyngeal level (Kelly–Paterson syndrome), and atrophic gastritis known to occur in iron-deficiency anemia in adults occurs only rarely, if ever, in adolescents.

Reduced *gastric acidity,* both under basal conditions and following histamine stimulation, has been demonstrated in iron-deficient children (17).

Iron-deficiency anemia per se may result in loss of blood from the gut. In this condition, infants have iron-deficiency anemia associated with *guaiac-positive stools.* Correction of the iron-deficiency anemia with iron reverses this process, and bleeding from the gut ceases. This bleeding from the gut is not diet related but is due to iron-deficiency anemia and is corrected by iron administration.

Iron-deficiency anemia may induce an *exudative enteropathy,* or "leaky gut" syndrome, with a loss of red cells, plasma proteins, albumin, immune globulins, copper, and calcium. This enteropathy can be completely corrected by iron therapy without any dietary change (18). It is caused by iron-deficiency anemia and aggravates existing iron deficiency.

A generalized *malabsorption syndrome* has also been demonstrated in iron-deficiency anemia (19, 20) consisting of impaired absorption of xylose, fat, and vitamin A. This enteropathy has been associated with varying degrees of chronic duodenitis and mucosal atrophy on duodenal biopsy and with the finding of blood loss from the gut, which aggravates the existing iron deficiency. After treatment with iron, most of these abnormalities revert to normal. They indicate a diffuse and reversible enteropathy in children as a result of iron-deficiency anemia.

Betanin, the red pigment found in beets, appears to be more efficiently absorbed in iron-deficient persons than in normal persons. The increased betanin absorption results in the occurrence of red urine, *beeturia,* in iron-deficient subjects given beet puree.

Decreased cytochrome oxidase activity in the gut epithelium of iron-deficient patients and animals has been demonstrated (21). Decreased disaccharidase activity has also been demonstrated in iron deficiency anemia (22).

Central Nervous System

Iron-deficiency anemia is associated with fatigue, weakness, lack of ability to concentrate, and irritability (23). Studies on intellectual function in iron-deficient children have purported to demonstrate varying adverse effects of anemia on one or more cognitive processes, and some authors have concluded that in iron-deficiency anemia there is a disturbance in attention and perception which compromises scholastic performance (24). Although this is not fully proven, the weight of evidence appears to favor it. The subjective response to iron therapy in anemic, iron-deficient patients often considerably precedes the rise in hemoglobin values.

Cardiovascular System

A reduction in hemoglobin concentration with resultant decrease in the oxygen-carrying capacity of the blood is associated with a compensatory increase in heart rate and cardiac output. Such changes are rarely detectable until the hemoglobin concentration has fallen to 7 g/dl or less. With increasing severity of anemia, cardiac enlargement and murmurs may develop and decompensation can occur. These features, however, are common to all severe anemias and are not specific for iron deficiency.

Musculoskeletal System

The correlation between anemia and physical capacity strongly suggests that the defect in iron deficiency is primarily one of reduced oxygen-carrying capacity of the blood because of its decreased content of hemoglobin. Available information indicates that physical endurance, activity, and manual-labor productivity are significantly curtailed in adults with hemoglobin values below 11 g/dl.

Cellular Metabolism

Red Cells (25).   In iron-deficiency anemia there is not only a decrease in hemoglobin synthesis but a profound effect on the overall metabolism of hemopoietic tissue.

Other Tissues.   Deficiencies in heme-containing enzymes (cytochrome C, cytochrome oxidase) and iron-dependent enzymes (succinic dehydrogenase, aconitase) have been demonstrated in the tissues of animals with latent iron deficiency (sideropenia without significant anemia).

Mitochondrial monoamine oxidase (MAO) is an enzyme sensitive to the state of body iron stores. It seems possible that at least a portion of the behavorial aberrations commonly attributed to iron deficiency may be caused by impaired MAO function and associated excesses of central nervous system (CNS) catechols.

Many other metabolic changes have been demonstrated in many tissues in iron-deficiency anemia. Table 7-12 summarizes the tissue effects of iron-deficiency anemia.

DIAGNOSIS

Table 7-13 summarizes the diagnostic test results in the investigation of iron-deficiency anemia. Anemia in the absence of other hematologic abnormalities is most probably due to iron deficiency. The presence of microcytosis (MCV as determined on the Coulter Model S < 70 μm^3) and hypochromia (MCHC $< 30\%$) are consistent with the diagnosis. The diagnosis is confirmed by a low serum iron, and elevated iron-binding capacity, and a transferrin saturation of 16% or less, a low serum ferritin, and absent bone marrow iron. The easiest and most reliable diagnostic criterion is the response of the anemia to iron. If iron is taken and the hemoglobin level does not increase in 3 weeks, the diagnosis of iron-deficiency anemia is probably erroneous unless bleeding has occurred. The characteristic diagnostic features are shown in Table 7-14.

In addition to making a diagnosis of iron-deficiency anemia, it is necessary to demonstrate its cause. The history should take into account all factors related to the development of iron deficiency. These should include a careful dietary history and consideration of all factors leading to blood loss. The most common site of bleeding is the bowel, and the most important investigation is examination of the stools for occult blood. If found, its cause should be established by examination of the stools for ova, rectal examination, sigmoidoscopy, barium enema, upper gastrointestinal series, and ^{99m}Tc pertechnetate scan for Meckel's diverticulum. Occasionally gastroscopy and colonoscopy are required. Negative guaiac tests occur, particularly if bleeding is intermittent, and for this reason occult bleeding should be tested for on at least five occasions when gastrointestinal bleeding is suspected. The guaiac test is only

Table 7-12. Tissue Effects of Iron Deficiency

Gastrointestinal tract
  Anorexia
    Increased proportion of low-weight percentiles
    Depression of growth
  Pica
  Atrophic glossitis
  Dysphagia
  Esophageal webs (Kelly-Paterson syndrome)
  Reduced gastric acidity
  "Leaky gut" syndrome
      Guaiac-positive stools
      Exudative enteropathy (protein, albumin, immune globulins, copper, calcium)
  Malabsorption syndrome
      Iron only
      Generalized malabsorption (xylose, fat, vitamin A, duodenojejunal mucosal atrophy)
  Beeturia
  Decreased cytochrome oxidase activity, succinic dehydrogenase and lactose

Central nervous system
  Irritability
  ? Lower IQ scores
  ? Decreased attentiveness, narrow attention span
  ? Significantly lower scholastic performance
  Breath-holding spells
  Papilledema

Cardiovascular system
  Increase in exercise and recovery heart rate and cardiac output
  Cardiac hypertrophy
  Increase in plasma volume
  Increased minute ventilation values
  Increased tolerance to digitalis

Musculoskeletal system
  Deficiency of myoglobin and cytochrome C
  Decreased physical performance
  Roentgenologic changes in bone
  Adverse effect on fracture healing

Cellular changes
  Red Cells:
    Ineffective erythropoiesis
    Decreased red cell survival (normal when injected into asplenic individuals)
    Increased autohemolysis
    Increased red cell rigidity

Table 7-12. *(continued)*

Cellular changes
  Red Cells *(continued)*
    Increased susceptibility to sulfhydryl inhibitors
    Decreased heme production
    Decreased globin and α-globin monomers to cell membrane
    Decreased glutathione peroxidase and catalase activity
      $\rightarrow$ Inefficient H_2O_2 detoxification
      $\rightarrow$ Greater susceptibility to H_2O_2 hemolysis
      $\rightarrow$ Oxidative damage to cell membrane
      $\rightarrow$ Increased cellular rigidity
    Increase in rate of glycolysis—glucose-6-phosphate dehydrogenase, 6-phosphogluconate dehydrogenase, 2,3-diphosphoglycerate (2,3-DPG) and glutathione
    Increase in NADH-methemoglobin reductase
    Increase in erythrocyte glutamic oxaloacetic transaminase (EGOT)
    Increase in free erythrocyte protoporphyrin
    Impairment of DNA and RNA synthesis in bone marrow cells
  Other tissues:
    Reduction in heme-containing enzymes (cytochrome C, cytochrome oxidase)
    Reduction in iron-dependent enzymes (succinic dehydrogenase, aconitase)
    Reduction in monoamine oxidase (MAO)
    Increased excretion of urinary norepinephrine
    ? Reduction in tyrosine hydroxylase (enzyme converting tyrosine to dihydroxyphenylalanine)
    Alterations in cellular growth, DNA, RNA, and protein
    Persistent deficiency of brain iron following short-term deprivation

Reduction in plasma zinc

Table 7-13. Diagnostic Test Results in Iron-Deficiency Anemia

Blood smear: hypochromic, microcytic red cells: MCV <70 μm³, MCH <27 pg, MCHC <30%

Bone marrow: delayed cytoplasmic maturation, decreased/absent stainable iron

Serum iron: decreased serum iron, increased iron-binding capacity, decreased transferrin saturation percentage

Plasma ferritin: decreased

Free erythrocyte protoporphyrin/hemoglobin ratio: elevated

Cobalt excretion test: increased excretion of ^{57}Co orally administered

Iron-absorption test: increased

Deferroxamine chelation test: iron excretion following injection correlates with iron stores

Therapeutic response to oral iron

Table 7-14.   Characteristics of Iron-Deficiency Anemia

Demonstrable cause of iron deficiency
Hypochromic-microcytic erythrocytes
Transferrin saturation of 16% or less
Low serum ferritin
Absence of bone marrow iron
Beneficial response to iron therapy:
  Reticulocytosis with peak 5–10 days after institution of therapy
  Reappearance of normochromic erythrocytes (dimorphic RBC population)
  Correction of anemia within 4 weeks

sensitive enough to pick up more than 5 ml of occult blood. Excessive uterine bleeding in menstruating females, epistaxis, renal blood loss (hematuria), and on rare occasions bleeding into the lung (idiopathic pulmonary hemosiderosis and Goodpasture's syndrome) may all be causes of iron-deficiency anemia. Bleeding into these areas requires specific investigations designed to identify the bleeding and determine its cause.

TREATMENT

The treatment of iron-deficiency anemia can be considered in two aspects: treatment of the individual patient and treatment of iron-deficiency anemia as a major public health problem. Successful management of the individual patient requires a thorough investigation of the cause of the negative iron balance resulting in iron deficiency, such as faulty diet, increased iron requirements due to rapid growth, or blood loss due to a structural gastrointestinal defect such as polyps or Meckel's diverticulum.

Nutritional Counseling

Most commonly, the history will reveal a dependence on foods notably poor in iron content, such as milk, cereals, and other carbohydrate foods. Often this situation will have developed unwittingly from the failure to understand the need for a well-balanced diet, particularly in the rapidly growing adolescent. Introduction of meat, vegetables, and fruit and supplementation by an iron preparation will usually suffice to correct the anemia.

Iron Medication

Simple iron salts are effective in correcting iron-deficiency anemia. Treatment with a soluble iron salt, preferably ferrous iron, corrects the deficiency promptly. Any form of ferrous iron, for example, ferrous gluconate, ferrous ascorbate, ferrous lactate, ferrous succinate, ferrous fumarate, or ferrous glycine sulfate, is effective. Ferric irons and heavily chelated iron should not be used as they are poorly and inefficiently absorbed. Vitamin supplementation or the addition of other heavy metals is unnecessary. Timed-release or enteric-coated products are not reliably absorbed; they may transport the iron past the duodenum and proximal jejunum where most iron absorption takes place. Side effects following iron medication include epigastric pain, nausea, diarrhea, and constipation. The side effects are related to the amount of elemental iron available for absorption and not to the type of preparation. Many preparations reputed to have a lower incidence of side effects also have a lower iron content or contain chelated iron, which has a lower therapeutic index.

Dosage and Mode of Administration

Since the percentage of metallic iron content is a fraction of the entire compound, iron should be prescribed with this in mind. Preparations available are suitably designated according to iron content.

Oral administration of iron usually results in the stool's becoming a deep black color because of the increased content of iron sulfides. The absence of this change may serve as a clue to irregular administration of the iron (26). Ingestion of liquid iron preparations may produce a black staining of the teeth. Brushing the teeth after each administration is of value in reducing this effect, although the staining is only temporary.

For adolescents, tablets of ferrous sulfate or ferrous gluconate are preferable to the concentrated liquid preparations. Gastric irritation, nausea, vomiting, and abdominal pain are less likely to occur if the tablets are taken with meals. Iron tablets are best taken 3 times daily at mealtime. Tablets of ferrous sulfate (0.2 g, 3 gr) or ferrous gluconate (0.3 g, 5 gr) given 3 times daily provide a daily total of 100 to 200 mg of elemental iron.

Full therapeutic doses of iron should be given for at least 6 to 8 weeks after the hemoglobin has been restored to normal levels. If oral therapy is withdrawn too soon, the iron stores will remain unreplenished and anemia will eventually recur (27). Serum ferritin, reflecting iron stores, rises significantly when oral treatment is continued for 2 months after attainment of a normal hemoglobin concentration.

Response to Oral Iron Therapy

Satisfactory response to iron may be heralded by an increase in appetite and improvement in disposition. A peak reticulocyte response is reached on the fifth to tenth day after institution of iron therapy, the reticulocyte increase being inversely proportional to the severity of the anemia. Following this the hemoglobin rises at an average of 0.25 to 0.4 g/dl per day, or a 1% per day rise in hematocrit reading during the first 7 to 10 days of therapy. Thereafter the hemoglobin rises at a slower rate, 0.1 to 0.15 g/dl per day. The magnitude of the response is related to the degree of anemia.

A substantial hemoglobin rise should be observed approximately 3 weeks after beginning iron therapy. Failure to achieve a level of at least 11 g/dl in this period with adequate iron therapy indicates that the diagnosis of anemia on a purely nutritional basis is to be questioned and suggests the continuation of an infectious process, underlying renal abnormality, continued blood loss, or impaired absorption.

Changes in mental status and appetite following iron therapy may occur within 48 to 72 hours (before a hematologic response occurs), suggesting that restoration of enzyme function is a more rapid process than correction of anemia.

Failure of Response to Oral Iron

When a patient fails to respond to oral iron the following reasons should be considered:

1. Failure or irregular administration of oral iron. Administration can be verified by change in stool color to gray-black or by testing stool for iron.
2. Inadequate iron dose.
3. Ineffective iron preparation.
4. Persistent or unrecognized blood loss, with the patient losing iron as fast as it is replaced.
5. Incorrect diagnosis.
6. Coexistent disease which interferes with absorption or utilization or iron, e.g., infection, malignant disease, hepatic or renal disease, concomitant deficiencies (vitamin B_{12}, folic acid, thyroid), associated lead poisoning.
7. Impaired gastrointestinal absorption, e.g., concurrent administration of large amounts of antacids (which bind iron) as treatment of peptic ulcer.

Parenteral Therapy

Iron-dextran complex for intramuscular use should be employed only under the following conditions:

1. Failure to take iron. Patient noncompliance.
2. Severe bowel disease (e.g., inflammatory bowel disease) associated with iron-deficiency anemia, in which the use of oral iron might aggravate the underlying disease of the gut.
3. Genuine intolerance to oral iron.
4. Chronic hemorrhage (e.g., hereditary telangiectasia, menorrhagia).
5. Acute diarrheal disorder in underprivileged populations with iron-deficiency anemia.

Iron-dextran is a high-molecular-weight complex of ferric hydroxide and dextran. The major amount of iron absorption following intramuscular injection occurs in 72 hours but at the end of 28 days some 10 to 50% of the dose may still remain at the site.

Iron-dextran complex for intramuscular use (Imferon) has proved a valuable adjunct to therapy. It is safe, effective, and well tolerated even in infants with a variety of acute illnesses, including acute diarrheal disorders. The total amount of iron needed to raise the hemoglobin level to normal and replenish stores is calculated as follows:

$$\frac{\text{Normal hemoglobin} - \text{initial hemoglobin}}{100} \times \text{blood volume (ml)} \times 3.4 \times 1.5$$

1. Normal hemoglobin: 14 to 15 g/dl at puberty.
2. Blood volume: 80 ml/kg or 40 ml/lb of body weight.
3. Multiplication by 3.4 converts grams of hemoglobin into milligrams of iron.
4. Factor 1.5 provides extra iron to replace depleted tissue stores.

Iron-dextran complex provides 50 mg elemental iron/ml. Once the total amount has been calculated it may be given in divided doses but should not be exceeded or repeated. Injections into the upper outer quadrant of the gluteus muscle are given through skin which has been displaced laterally prior to the injection to prevent superficial staining. Untoward reactions are rare. Occasionally fever lasting 24 to 48 hours occurs. Less commonly staining of the skin occurs when there is leakage beneath the skin because the iron was not given deep enough into the muscle or because of "streaking" along the path of withdrawal of the needle. In rare cases local or generalized reactions, angioneurotic edema, and recurrent arthralgia occur. The carcinogenic risks of iron-dextran complex in laboratory animals appear to have no relevance in clinical medicine (28).

If hemoglobin values do not rise at least 2 g in 3 weeks, other possible causes of anemia should be considered, and more iron should not be administered. Failure to respond requires further hematologic investigation. The use of iron-dextran complex intravenously is dangerous and should be avoided, since this can cause anaphylactic reactions.

A new preparation for intramuscular use has recently been introduced (29, 30). This is a sterile aqueous solution of iron-polysorbitol-gluconic acid complex (Ferastral-Astra, Sweden). The preparation appears to be a safe, effective iron preparation. After intramuscular injection it is absorbed exclusively via the lymphatic route. After 48 hours 75% of the dose is absorbed, and after 10 days 82%.

As with other intramuscular iron preparations, staining at the site of injection may occur with this product, especially in cases where the solution is accidentally administered into the superficial tissues. Staining is of a transient type, disappearing after a few weeks or months. The local inflammatory reaction is slight. Side effects of a general type have occurred in rare cases. There have been complaints of nausea and dizziness in occasional cases.

Treatment of Anemia as a Public Health Problem

Iron deficiency is the only known vitamin or mineral deficiency still prevalent in an era in which such diseases as scurvy, rickets, and pellagra have become rarities. The Food and Nutrition Board of the National Academy of Sciences has proposed to increase iron supplementation in flour from the present level of 13.0 to 16.5 mg/lb to between 40 and 60 mg/lb (31). This should assure an adequate iron supply for adolescents and postpubertal females. The most appropriate food selected for iron enrichment may vary in different parts of the world and in different ethnic and social groups. At present such supplemented food staples are not in general use and efforts to identify and develop suitable vehicles for enrichment are essential if optimal iron nutrition is to be assured.

Experience with nutritional deficiencies of sufficient magnitude to constitute public health problems has demonstrated that they can be managed through public health measures. The addition of vitamin D to milk has virtually prevented the development of nutritional rickets in children in the United States and has eliminated rickets as a public health problem. Judicious enrichment programs involving vitamin C have also eliminated scurvy as a public health problem. Likewise, judicious enrichment programs with iron should eliminate iron-deficiency anemia.

REFERENCES

1. D. Schachter et al.: *Am. J. Physiol.*, **198**, 609 (1960); **203**, 73 (1962); **207**, 893 (1964).
2. M. S. Wheby et al., *J. Clin. Invest.*, **42**, 1007 (1963); **43**, 1433 (1964); *Blood*, **22**, 416 (1963); *N. Engl. J. Med.*, **271**, 1391 (1964).
3. T. H. Bothwell et al., *J. Lab. Clin. Med.*, **51**, 24 (1958).
4. M. Layrisse et al., *Blood*, **33**, 430 (1969).

5.   C. V. Moore et al., *J. Clin. Invest.*, **23**, 755 (1944).

6.   I. M. Sharpe et al., *J. Nutr.*, **41**, 433 (1950).

7.   M. J. Murray and N. Stein, *J. Lab. Clin. Med.*, **70**, 673 (1967); *Proc. Soc. Exp. Biol. Med.*, **133**, 183 (1970).

8.   P. S. David, et al., *Lancet*, **2**, 1431 (1966).

9.   P. M. Smith, *Lancet*, **2**, 1143 (1968).

10.   M. S. Wheby et al., *Gastroenterology*, **42**, 310 (1962).

11.   H. A. Pearson et al., *J.A.M.A.*, **215**, 1982 (1971).

12.   P. Lanzkowsky, *Iron Deficiency Anemia: A Public Health Problem*, Mead Johnson, Evanston, Ind., 1975.

13.   C. T. Greenwood and D. P. Richardson, *Wld. Rev. Nutr. Diet*, **33**, (1979).

14.   W. A. Daniel, E. G. Gaines, and D. L. Bennet, *J. Pediat.*, **86**, 288 (1975).

15.   J. M. Judisch et al., *Pediatrics*, **37**, 987 (1966).

16.   P. Lanzkowsky, *Arch. Dis. Child.*, **34**, 140 (1959).

17.   S. Chosh et al., *Am. J. Dis. Child.*, **123**, 14 (1972).

18.   P. Lanzkowsky, "Iron Metabolism and Iron-Deficiency Anemia," in D. R. Miller and H. A. Pearson, Eds., *Smith's Blood Diseases of Infancy and Children*, Mosby, St. Louis, 1978.

19.   J. L. Naiman et al., *Pediatrics*, **33**, 83 (1964).

20.   D. K. Guha et al., *Arch. Dis. Child.*, **43**, 239 (1968).

21.   P. R. Dallman et al., *Pediatrics*, **39**, 863 (1967).

22.   P. Lanzkowsky et al., *Ped. Res.*, **12**, 468 (1978).

23.   P. Lanzkowsky, *Acta. Paediatr. Scand.*, **50**, 25 (1961).

24.   E. Pollitt and R. L. Leibel, *J. Pediatr.*, **88**, 372 (1976).

25.   L. G. Macdougall et al., *J. Pediatr.*, **76**, 660 (1970).

26.   N. J. Smith, *J. Pediatr.*, **53**, 37 (1958).

27.   C. H. Smith et al., "Iron Metabolism in Infants and Children: Serum Iron and Iron-Binding Protein: Diagnostic and Therapeutic Implications", in S. Z. Levine, Ed., *Advances in Pediatrics*, Vol. 5, Year Book, Chicago, 1952, p. 195.

28.   P. Lanzkowsky, *S. Afr. Med. J.*, **34**, 351 (1960).

29.   K. Domeij et al., *Scand. J. Haematol.*, **32**, 21 (1977).

30.   B. Swedberg, *Scand. J. Haematol.*, **32**, 260 (1977).

31.   Council on Foods and Nutrition, *J.A.M.A.*, **220**, 855 (1972).

8

Nutritional Role of Zinc and Effects of Deficiency

HAROLD H. SANDSTEAD, M.D.

United States Department of Agriculture, Science and Education Administration, Grand Forks Human Nutrition Research Center, Grand Forks, North Dakota

The essentiality of zinc for higher animals was established in 1934 by Todd et al. (1) who found that zinc deprivation in rats severely retarded growth. Subsequently, it was reported that blood and tissue zinc levels were decreased in human malnutrition (2). The occurrence of human zinc deficiency was believed unlikely until Tucker and Salmon (3) reported that porcine parakeratosis was responsive to zinc, and Vallee et al. (4) described conditioned zinc deficiency in humans with alcoholic cirrhosis. Soon after, dietary zinc deficiency conditioned by parasitism or geophagia was reported in adolescents from Egypt (5, 6) and Iran (7).

BIOCHEMICAL FUNCTION

Zinc is required for the activity of more than 70 enzymes in various species. It is required for the activity of at least one enzyme in each of the six categories of the International Union Biochemists System of Enzyme Nomenclature (8). Its participation in so many metabolic processes provides explanations for some of the effects of deficiency. For example, depressed activity of alcohol dehydrogenase associated with zinc deficiency (9) impairs dark adaptation and might contribute to the testicular atrophy observed in some zinc-deficient subjects (10). The essentiality of zinc for activity of thymidine kinase (11), DNA polymerase (12), and reverse transcriptase (13) of various species provides a possible explanation for the impaired cell replication of zinc-deficient animals. The suppressed activity of RNA polymerase (14, 15) may explain the impaired protein synthesis (16–18) observed in zinc-deficient animals. It seems possible that the depressed pancreatic carboxypeptidase A activity that occurs in zinc-deficient experimental animals (19) impairs digestion of protein and thus contributes to depressed utilization of dietary protein (20).

ZINC DEFICIENCY IN EXPERIMENTAL ANIMALS

Among the earliest effects of zinc deficiency in animals are anorexia and cyclic feeding (21), severe impairment in metabolic efficiency, and depressed growth (22). Later dermatitis (23), depressed immune function (24–26), impaired healing (27), suppressed gonadal function (28,29), and gonadal atrophy (30) occur.

Zinc deficiency early in pregnancy produces severe teratologic abnormalities in embryos (31). During parturition zinc deficiency results in prolonged labor, hemorrhage, and maternal death (28, 32). Deficiency during the critical period of brain development impairs maturation (33), cell division (34, 35), and dendritic arborization (35). Long-term sequellae of zinc deficiency during the period of rapid brain growth include behavioral abnormalities in both rats (36–40) and monkeys (41, 42). Recent work suggests that zinc is required for synaptic function (43) and that acute deficiency increases brain norepinephrine (44).

ZINC METABOLISM

The absorption of zinc by the intestine is homeostatically controlled. Studies in rats have shown there is an increase in percent true absorption and true utilization when suboptimal amounts are fed (22). When diets contain liberal amounts of zinc, the true absorption by rats is about 25% and utilization is about 18%. Perfusion studies in rats suggest that approximately three times as much zinc is absorbed in the ilium as in the duodenum and the jejunum (45). However, other studies in animals (46, 47) and humans (48), in which different techniques were used, suggest that under usual conditions maximal absorption occurs in the duodenum. The absorption of zinc is an active process which is suppressed by anaerobic conditions (49). It appears that prostaglandins E_2 and F_2 may mediate absorption and excretion. In rats PGE_2 substantially increased intestinal absorption and liver accumulation of zinc, while PGF_2 facilitated its excretion into the intestinal lumen (49). A product of vitamin B_6-dependent tryptophan metabolism, picolinic acid, present in pancreatic juice facilitates the uptake of zinc by intestinal mucosal cells (50). Within intestinal mucosal cells, the movement of zinc from the mucosa to the serosa seems to be regulated by metallothionein, a sulfur-rich protein whose synthesis is induced by zinc (51, 52). Much of the zinc entering the cells is complexed by this protein and may be returned to the intestinal lumen in the process of cell turnover. In some experiments, the induction of metallothionein by zinc has been associated with an increase in transport of zinc across the intestinal mucosa (53). Entry of zinc into portal blood is believed to occur by formation of a complex with transferrin (54).

The uptake of zinc from foods is related to its availability. When animal protein sources are increased, the absorption of zinc is increased (55, 56). It seems possible the picolinic acid and/or other facilitating ligands, present in such foods, are partly responsible for the greater uptake. Amino acids, such as histidine, cysteine, and cystine will form complexes with zinc and facilitate its absorption (57). Protein deficiency impairs zinc absorption (55). Supplementation of protein-deficient diets with tryptophan or its metabolite picolinic acid will restore zinc absorption (58). Substances in plants, including phytate (myoinositol hexaphosphate) (59), hemicellulose (60), and lignin (61), as well as phytate–amino acid compounds produced during food processing (62) and products of the Maillard reaction (63), are potential inhibitors of zinc absorption. If these are present in diets in large amounts, the availability of zinc may be significantly compromised. For example, when volunteers were fed a diet prepared exclusively of fruits and vegetables the absorption of zinc from the diet was low (64). In another study the addition of black beans or tortillas to oysters significantly decreased the absorption of zinc from the oysters (65). In some instances a food rich in inhibitors of zinc absorption may be a better source of zinc than a food nearly free of inhibitors. For example, the net amount of [65]Zn absorbed from whole wheat bread was greater than the amount absorbed from unenriched white bread (56). The zinc content of the whole wheat bread was so much greater than that of the white bread, that the net absorption of zinc from the whole wheat bread was greater. Nondietary substances that may inhibit zinc absorption include ferrous iron (66) and clay (67).

Zinc excretion occurs primarily via the gastrointestinal tract (68). Our studies indicate that the zinc intake of persons eating mixed Western diets is the major factor influencing the level of fecal zinc ($n = 161, r^2 = 0.77, p < 0.0001$). Losses across the intestinal wall may be substantial. In rats this process is stimulated by PGF_2 (49). Studies in bovines indicate that losses via pancreatic secretion may also be large (69). Although urinary excretion of zinc is relatively small, our studies indicate the level of zinc in urine is influenced primarily by the interaction of dietary nitrogen and phosphorus ($n = 161, r^2 = 0.16, p < 0.0001$). Usual amounts lost in urine range from 300 to 600 μg/day (70). Persons severely depleted of zinc may excrete less than 100 μg/day in urine (71, 72). Hyperzincuria may occur in association with severe liver injury secondary to alcoholism (73) or hepatitis (74), nephrotic syndrome (75), histidinuria (76), and subsequent to infusion of certain amino acid mixtures used in total parenteral alimentation, apparently due to the presence of Maillard products (77).

Surface losses of zinc are similar to those in urine under mild environmental conditions (78). When the environmental temperature is high, the surface loss of zinc may exceed 1 mg/liter (79).

Zinc is transported in the blood plasma primarily as a loose complex with albumin. Most of the remaining one-third of plasma zinc is present in alpha-2-macroglobulin metalloprotein (80). A small amount of plasma zinc is complexed with amino acids and possibly with picolinic acid.

Under usual conditions, there is a circadian variation in plasma zinc, deviating about 7% around the mean (81). "Normal" fasting morning plasma values range from about 70 to 125 μg/dl in various laboratories (82). Reported mean values range from about 85 to 110 μg/dl. Subsequent to eating, plasma zinc often decreases. An increase in plasma zinc occurs if a food rich in zinc, such as oysters, is eaten (65). If foods are rich in inhibitors of zinc absorption, the postprandial increase in plasma zinc does not occur. When the protein content of a diet is high an exaggerated postprandial decrease in plasma zinc may occur (56). The cause of this phenomenon has not been defined.

Erythrocyte zinc levels range from about 10 to 14 μg/ml (83). Much of the red cell zinc is present in carbonic anhydrase and superoxide dismutase.

Tracer amounts of oral zinc chloride are rapidly absorbed, the peak value occurring at about 2 hours (48). The first 24 hours after absorption 40% of the tracer is present in the liver (84). Over the subsequent several days, the amount of tracer decreases until about 25% is present after 5 days. The uptake of zinc by the liver is stimulated by ACTH (85), Leukocyte Endogenous Mediator, and endotoxin (86). Zinc taken up by the liver induces the synthesis of metallothionein with which it forms a complex (87). Zinc not complexed with metallothionein probably participates in the synthesis of acute phase proteins through mechanisms previously alluded to. Subsequently, much of the zinc taken up in response to these stimuli is excreted or redistributed to other tissues. The turnover of zinc-metallothionein complexes is relatively slow (88). It is unresolved whether formation of zinc metallothionein complex represents a detoxification mechanism, a storage mechanism, or both.

Concentrations of zinc in tissues vary widely. For example, skeletal muscle contains 50 μg/g, while liver and heart contain about 30 μg/g. Levels in prostate and bone are high, exceeding 100 μg/g. The whole body concentration of zinc is about 33 μg/g. Concentrations in retina, hippocampus, and epididymis are much higher than in other tissues (70).

The turnover of zinc within the body is slow, the half-life exceeding 250 days (89). Under usual circumstances zinc in bone exchanges little with soft tissue. For practical purposes, therefore, bone zinc is not a readily available store for times of increased need. On the other hand, when dietary calcium is low and in circumstances where bone calcium is being mobilized, bone zinc is also released and is available to the soft tissues (90). Under circumstances of stress, there is mobilization of zinc from peripheral tissues to the liver (86). Redistribution of zinc in the body apparently also occurs during healing (91, 92). An increased local need is believed to be the stimulus.

ASSESSMENT OF ZINC STATUS

At present, there is no single, unequivocal index for measurement of zinc status of humans (93). Plasma zinc represents the most readily available and easily analyzed zinc pool. However, under circumstances of deficiency, plasma zinc may not reliably reflect depletion (72, 94). A finding of low plasma zinc is presumptive evidence of impaired zinc nutriture, if a redistribution of zinc caused by an acute stimulus can be ruled out. On the other hand, normal·plasma levels may be found even though the patient is zinc depleted. Long-standing zinc depletion may result in a decrease in erythrocyte zinc. Zinc content of leukocytes is depressed in zinc deficiency. Levels of zinc in hair may be decreased in patients with chronic moderate depletion (95). On the other hand, patients with severe zinc deficiency may display normal or increased levels (96). In such patients the level of hair zinc may initially decrease and then return to normal with repletion. Urinary excretion of zinc is significantly decreased when dietary zinc is severely restricted (72). As the depletion continues patients display a progressively more severe negative zinc balance and urine levels increase, but remain in the low range (94). A finding of very low urinary zinc, less than 100 $\mu g/g$, is presumptive evidence of severe zinc depletion. Fecal zinc is also low when dietary zinc is severely restricted. As deficiency becomes more severe, the losses in feces increase (94).

Zinc nutriture can also be evaluated by measurements of physiological and biochemical function. For example, serum alkaline phosphatase may be decreased in severe zinc deficiency (97), and impaired dark adaptation can reflect impaired zinc nutriture (10). Impaired immunity occurs in association with zinc deficiency (96, 98−100). Impaired taste and smell acuity may signify zinc deficiency (10, 76, 95), as may increased bleeding time and depressed platelet aggregation in response to adenosine diphosphate, collagen, or arachidonic acid (101).

Patient response to a therapeutic trial with zinc may in some instances be the only conclusive way to establish a diagnosis of zinc deficiency.

ZINC LEVELS IN FOODS AND DIETS

Knowledge of the levels of zinc in foods is incomplete. The United States Department of Agriculture has published a preliminary compilation of the zinc content of selected foods and the amounts of zinc in commonly consumed portions (Table 8-1) (102). The estimated contribution of the various food groups to the dietary intake of zinc of persons in the United States has also been published (Table 8-2) (103). The best sources of zinc are meat, poultry, and seafoods. Levels in unrefined cereals are fairly high. Refinement typically removes most of the zinc. When meat, fish, and poultry are not included in the diet, legumes are an important source. Levels of zinc in dairy products are relatively low.

Zinc is most available for absorption from meat, fish, and poultry. Availability from cow milk and cheese appears to be less than from meat (104). For reasons noted previously the availability of zinc from plant materials is generally poor compared to meat.

Table 8-1.   Zinc Content of Common Household Portions of Selected Foods (102)

Food	Portions	Zinc (mg)
Fish, light poultry meat, shellfish (except crab and oyster)	3 oz.	<2.0
Poultry liver, dark chicken meat	3 oz.	2.0/3.0
Pork, veal, crab, dark turkey meat, ground beef (77% lean)	3 oz.	3.0/4.0
Beef liver, beef	3 oz.	4.0/5.0
Oyster	3 oz.	>5.0
Egg (whole)	1	0.5
Peanut butter	2 Tbsp.	0.9
Mature dried beans, lentils, chickpeas, split peas (boiled, drained)	½ cup	0.9/1.0
Cow peas, black eyed peas (boiled, drained)	½ cup	1.5
Milk: Whole fluid	1 cup	0.9
Canned, evaporated	½ cup	1.0
Dried, nonfat, instant	⅓ cup	1.0
Ice cream	1½ cup	1.0
Cheddar cheese	3 slices (1½ oz.)	1.6
Cooked oatmeal	1 cup	1.2
Cooked whole wheat cereal	1 cup	1.2
Wheat flakes	1 oz.	0.6
Bran flakes (40%)	1 oz.	1.0
Wheat germ (toasted)	1 Tbsp.	0.9
Corn flakes	1 oz.	0.08
Cooked corn meal	1 cup	0.3
White wheat bread	1 slice	0.2
Whole wheat bread	1 slice	0.5
Cooked brown rice (hot)	1 cup	1.2
Cooked white rice (hot)	1 cup	0.8
Precooked white rice (hot)	1 cup	0.4

DIETARY ZINC REQUIREMENTS

Requirements for zinc have been estimated both factorially (105) and by balance studies (106). Provisional dietary requirements based on factorial calculations were published in 1973 (107) (Table 8-3). These estimates included an adjustment for differences in availability for intestinal absorption caused by the presence of plant materials in the

Table 8-2. Contribution of Foods to Dietary Intake of Zinc (103)

Food Group	mg/kg As Purchased	mg Consumed/ Person/Day	% of Total Food Intake
Milk, cheese, ice cream	4.3	2.5	20
Meat, poultry, fish	18.6	5.5	43
Dry beans, peas, nuts	24.7	0.5	4
Eggs	12.7	0.6	5
Dark green and deep yellow vegetables	2.8	0.1	1
Citrus fruit, tomatoes	1.8	0.3	2
Potatoes	2.4	0.3	2
Other vegetables, fruit	2.0	0.7	6
Cereal, pasta	16.3	0.8	7
Flour, mixes	2.8	0.1	1
Bread	7.2	0.6	5
Other bakery products	6.0	0.4	3
Fats, oils	1.8	0.1	1
Sugar, sweets	0.6	0	0
Total food		12.5	100

diet. Recent studies suggest that requirements are also related to the level of dietary protein and phosphorus. The Recommended Dietary Allowances for zinc (Table 8-4) do not provide for wide variations in zinc availability or for effects of other nutrients on zinc requirements (108).

Information on infant requirements for zinc is limited. It appears that levels in cow milk are insufficient for young infants, whereas levels in human milk are more likely to be adequate (113, 114). Total amounts of zinc in these two milks are similar. Therefore the greater adequacy of human milk is believed to be caused by the presence of a facilitator of zinc absorption. Picolinic acid has been suggested to be such a facilitator (115), as has citrate (116). There is controversy whether one or both of these ligands facilitate zinc absorption from human milk. It is evident that an intake of 0.6 mg/Zn/kg is inadequate for preterm infants fed human milk (117) and that negative zinc balance and decreasing bone zinc may be evident for many weeks (118). Similarly, mature term infants may require higher levels of zinc than are present in mature human milk. It seems likely that the high levels of zinc in colostrum represent an important source of zinc for the newborn (119). Enrichment of cow milk formula to a level of about 5 mg/Zn/liter was sufficient to support greater growth in male infants (113). It appears that feeding

Table 8-3. Provisional Dietary Requirements for Zinc in Relation to Estimates of Retention, Losses, and Availability (107)[a]

Age	Peak Daily Retention (mg)	Urinary Excretion (mg)	Sweat Excretion (mg)	Total Required (mg)	Milligrams Necessary in Daily Diet if Content of Available Zinc Is:		
					10%	20%	40%
Infants:							
0–4 months	0.35	0.4	0.5	1.25	12.5	6.3	3.1
5–12 months	0.2	0.4	0.5	1.1	11.0	5.5	2.8
Males:							
1–10 years	0.2	0.4	1.0	1.6	16.0	8.0	4.0
11–17 years	0.8	0.5	1.5	2.8	28.0	14.0	7.0
18 years plus	0.2	0.5	1.5	2.2	22.0	11.0	5.5
Females:							
1–9 years	0.15	0.4	1.0	1.55	15.5	7.8	3.9
10–13 years	0.65	0.5	1.5	2.65	26.5	13.3	6.6
14–16 years	0.2	0.5	1.5	2.2	22.0	11.0	5.5
17 years plus	0.2	0.5	1.5	2.2	22.0	11.0	5.5
Pregnant women:							
0–20 weeks	0.55	0.5	1.5	2.55	25.5	12.8	6.4
20–30 weeks	0.9	0.5	1.5	2.9	29.0	14.5	7.3
30–40 weeks	1.0	0.5	1.5	3.0	30.0	15.0	7.5
Lactating women:	3.45	0.5	1.5	5.45	54.5	27.3	13.7

[a]The above estimates were based on the assumption that the fat-free tissue concentration of zinc in man is approximately 30 μg/g (109). This figure is equivalent to 2.0 g of zinc in the soft tissues of an adult male and 1.2 g in the soft tissues of an adult female, as determined from lean body mass (110). The zinc requirement at various ages was determined from the change in lean body mass with age. Bone zinc was not included in these calculations, because zinc in bone is relatively sequestered from the metabolically active pool of body zinc. The zinc content of sweat is based on an assumed zinc surface loss of 1 mg/liter (79). The estimated requirement for lactation is based on a zinc content in milk of 5 mg/liter (111) and a daily milk secretion of 650 ml. The urinary excretion of zinc is based on reported levels (67,112).

Table 8-4.   Recommended Dietary Allowance for Zinc (108)

Infants		Children	Males	Females	Pregnant	Lactating
Age: 0−0.5; 0.5−1.0		1−10	11−51+	11−51+		
(years)						
Zinc: 3	5	10	15	15	20	25
(mg)						

cow milk, unenriched cow milk formula, or formula prepared from soybeans may result in impaired zinc nutriture in some infants (114, 120).

Studies in young children suggest that an intake of 7 to 8 mg of readily available dietary zinc is adequate for growth (121). An increased intake of dietary protein had a positive effect on zinc retention. For example, when children were fed 50 g of protein and 7 mg of zinc daily, zinc retention was 2 mg/day. When they were fed 25 g/day of protein and 5 mg/day of zinc, they retained less than 1 mg/day.

The zinc requirement of children entering adolescence is greater than of children prior to adolescence (105). The principal cause is the accelerated growth that occurs at this time. Regression analysis of balance data suggested a requirement of about 11 mg/day by adolescent females fed 11.5−14 mg/day of Zn with 8 g of dietary nitrogen (122). When losses due to sweat and menses were included, the estimated requirement was 12.3 mg/day before menarche, and 11.9 mg/day after menarche. Factorial estimates of zinc requirements of adolescent males indicate that the maximum requirement occurs between 12 and 13 years (105).

The dietary zinc requirements of adult men fed mixed Western diets have been estimated by metabolic balance (106). When the data from 161 30-day metabolic balance studies at the Grand Forks Human Nutrition Research Center were evaluated by multiple stepwise regression analysis of the predictors, zinc balance, calcium intake, phosphorus intake, nitrogen intake, and the interactions among these predictors, it was found that 83% of the variance in requirement was explained ($p <$ 0.0001) by the following equation when balance was in equilibrium:

$$\text{Requirement} = -7.59 + 0.23 \, (\text{balance}) + 9.60p + 0.81N - 0.30 \, (p \times N)$$

The zinc requirements when diets contain four levels of dietary protein and phosphorus calculated from this equation are shown in Table 8-5. Note that zinc requirements are increased when both dietary phosphorus and protein are high, and that dietary phosphorus has the greatest effect on the requirement. The addition of surface losses of zinc to the requirements shown in Table 8-5 will increase the requirement of persons living in temperate environments by about 0.5 mg/day (78). In regions where temperatures are high the increase may substantially exceed 1.0 mg/day (79).

Factorial calculations suggest that zinc requirements are substantially increased during pregnancy (107). An estimated 750 μg/day retention appears to be needed during the latter half of pregnancy (105). In young teenagers the requirement is probably even greater because the mother is still growing.

ZINC DEFICIENCY IN HUMANS

Zinc deficiency may occur in persons of all ages. Its occurrence is related to the quantity and availability of zinc in the diet and the balance between factors that interfere with zinc absorption or cause increased zinc loss and factors that facilitate zinc absorption and retention.

Zinc deficiency related to diet was first characterized by Prasad et al. (5, 6, 79, 123) in adolescent Egyptian village boys with dwarfism and hypogonadism. The causes of the deficiency were a diet predominantly of unleavened bread, rich in dietary fiber and phytate, and very low in meat and other animal products, and associated conditioning factors

Table 8-5. Relationship of Dietary Zinc Requirement (mg/day) to Dietary Protein and Phosphorus Intake of Men Fed Mixed Western Diets

Protein (g):	40	60	80	100
Phosphorus				
1000 (mg)	5.27	6.91	8.54	10.17
	(2.48–8.07[a]	(4.11–9.70)	(5.74–11.33)	(7.38–12.96)
1500	9.11	10.27	11.42	12.57
	(6.32–11.91)	(7.47–13.06)	(8.62–14.21)	(9.78–15.36)
2000	12.95	13.63	14.30	14.97
	(10.16–15.75)	(10.83–16.42)	(11.50–17.09)	(12.18–17.76)
2500	16.79	16.99	17.18	17.37
	(14.00–19.59)	(14.19–19.78)	(14.38–19.97)	(14.58–20.16)

[a]95% confidence interval.

including blood loss from hookworm and/or schistosomiasis infection and a high environmental temperature. Subsequent to treatment with zinc the boys displayed accelerated growth and sexual maturation (124). Prasad et al. (125) had previously reported similar patients from Iran. The principal conditioning factor in those patients was geophagia. The more severely affected Egyptian patients with Prasad's syndrome had physical findings and laboratory indices similar to those of patients with hypopituitarism (124, 126). Abnormal indices of zinc metabolism included low zinc in plasma, erythrocytes, hair, urine, and sweat; an accelerated disappearance of ^{65}Zn tracer from the peripheral blood; and increased body retention of the tracer. Subsequently the description of Prasad's syndrome was confirmed by others working in Iran and shown to occur in females (7).

Patients with the appearance of Prasad's syndrome have been reported from Turkey (127), Morocco, Portugal (67), the United States (128), and China (129). It is highly likely that dwarfism attributed in the past to hookworm (13) was, in fact, due to zinc deficiency.

Zinc deficiency also occurs in patients with severe protein-calorie malnutrition (98, 99, 131). In addition to contributing to growth failure, the deficiency causes atrophy of the thymus gland and is, in part, responsible for increased susceptibility to infection (99).

Less severe zinc deficiency occurs in school children in the Middle East. Iranian school boys with retarded growth and delayed sexual maturation have been shown to respond to zinc (132). School boys from an Egyptian oasis where hookworm and schistosomiasis do not occur were found to have low plasma zinc with delayed growth and maturation (133). Without the benefit of zinc therapy these boys experienced growth and sexual maturation (134). Their final stature was substantially below that of ethnically similar, more economically advantaged countrymen. In view of these findings from the Middle East it seems possible that short stature commonly observed among the poor of the region is in part related to widespread zinc deficiency. This interpretation is probably relevant to economically deprived populations throughout the world. Their high intakes of cereals, low intakes of meat, as well as the frequent occurrence of conditioning factors including infectious diseases and parasitism support this hypothesis.

Application of the above hypothesis to the risk of specific groups to zinc deficiency suggests that pregnant women are among the most at risk. Findings from Turkey indicate that poor women display lower plasma zinc levels during pregnancy (135). Because fetal rats exposed to zinc deficiency early in gestation display severe teratology (136, 137), these findings lend support to the hypothesis that the higher incidence of congenital malformations among infants of the Middle East is, in part, related to poor maternal zinc nutriture (138). Also supportive is the frequency of congenital malformations in infants of women with acrodermatitis enteropathica (139, 140).

Dietary zinc deficiency also occurs in industrialized countries. For example, growth failure and hypogeusia responsive to zinc has been reported in middle income preschool children from Denver, Colorado (95). The discovery was based on the finding of low concentrations of zinc in hair in some infants and children, and demonstrating a therapeutic response of the symptoms to zinc therapy. The major factor in the occurrence of the deficiency was poor food selection.

Other evidence consistent with zinc deficiency among children in the United States is the finding of an inverse association between growth rate and plasma zinc of inner-city children and the association between restricted family income and low plasma zinc in children in the Baltimore area (141, 142). The finding of a low zinc content in diets typical of poor children from the southeastern United States is additional evidence (105). If the zinc in these diets was only 20−30% available for absorption, the diets were inadequate to provide the factorially calculated requirement (107). Further evidence of zinc deficiency among children is the association between growth failure and low plasma and hair zinc in Denver children who were participating in a "Head Start" program (143).

Limited data suggest that dietary zinc deficiency occurs in some adolescents and young adults in the United States. The zinc content of self-selected diets of midwestern teenage girls and college women who were eating in a cafeteria was found to range from 4.8 to 47.0 mg/day (144). The high intakes were probably related to inclusion of liver in the diet. Comparison of the intakes with a factorial estimate of the zinc requirement suggested that about 20% of the women may have had deficient intake (105). Observations on Scandinavian teenagers with acne vulgaris suggest that some of them had not consumed adequate zinc. Zinc supplementation was followed by improvement in the acne (145−147).

Zinc nutriture may also be deficient in some pregnant women from industrial societies. Under usual circumstances plasma zinc concentrations decrease during pregnancy (148−151). An association between abnormal delivery and congenital malformations with low plasma zinc at midpregnancy or earlier has been reported from Sweden (151). As yet, confirmatory findings have not been reported.

The relation of plasma zinc to outcome of pregnancy is not entirely clear. Midpregnancy measurements of multiple indices of nutrition and other factors affecting outcome of pregnancy indicate that zinc is one of 13 nutritional indices that together accounted for about 20% of the variance in fetal growth in a test population of 250 women with uncomplicated pregnancies. When combined with other predictors of outcome, 65% of the variance in fetal growth could be explained (152). A surprising finding in this study was that plasma zinc was one of several indices that was elevated at midpregnancy in women who subsequently had small babies. Women with large babies had lower levels of plasma zinc along with lower levels of certain other nutrients. Hemoconcentration of maternal blood was associated with small babies in this population, presumably accounting for the elevated plasma zinc.

Evidence of dietary zinc deficiency has also been identified in elderly persons in the United States (153–155). Many persons living in institutions, or participating in congregate feeding programs, were found to consume less than two-thirds of the recommended dietary allowance for zinc. Hypogeusia was not uncommon and at least 10% had hair zinc concentrations less than 100 μg/g. In one study, 11% had hair zinc concentrations less than 70 μg/g and serum zinc levels less than 70 μg/dl. A variety of factors are probably responsible for these findings. They include the limitation in food choices caused by economic deprivation, anorexia associated with social isolation and depression, mechanical difficulties in masticating food, and inappropriate selection of foods. Indirect evidence of zinc deficiency among elderly persons and others is the occurrence of zinc-responsive impaired healing.

Improved healing subsequent to zinc therapy implies previous poor zinc nutriture. Studies in animals have shown that improved healing of wounds subsequent to zinc supplementation only occurs when zinc deficiency is present (27). The beneficial effect of zinc on healing of zinc-deficient humans has been established by carefully controlled double-blind studies (156, 157).

CONDITIONED ZINC DEFICIENCY

The most severe instances of zinc deficiency occur in association with conditioning factors that impair absorption of zinc or increase zinc excretion. Some diseases and other conditions with which zinc deficiency may be associated are listed in Table 8-6. Infants with acrodermatitis enteropathica display some of the most severe manifestations of zinc deficiency (158). Signs of deficiency usually begin after the infants have been weaned from breast milk. They include a vesiculobullous hyper-

Table 8-6.   Some Potential Causes of Zinc Deficiency

Primary Deficiency
  Low dietary intake
    Protein-energy deficient diets
  Low availability of dietary zinc
    Diets very high in phytate, dietary fiber, and Maillard products
      Iatrogenic
    Inadequate parenteral or enteral alimentation
Conditioned Deficiency
  Genetic and congenital defects
    Acrodermatitis enteropathica
    Thalassemia
    Sickle cell disease
    Cystic fibrosis
    Coeliac sprue
    Hypogammaglobulinemia
    Porphyria
    Down's syndrome
    Diabetes mellitus
  Malabsorption syndromes
    Pancreatic insufficiency
    Biliary obstruction
    Gastrectomy (partial or total)
    Jejunoileostomy
    Intestinal diverticuli and blind loops
    Tropical sprue
    Coeliac sprue
    Cystic fibrosis
  Protein losing enteropathies
  Inflammatory diseases of the bowel
    Crohn's disease
    Ulcerative colitis
  Liver disease
    Hepatitis
    Cirrhosis
  Renal disease
    Nephrotic syndrome
    Chronic renal failure
  Exfoliative dermatitis
  Neuropsychiatric disease
    Anorexia nervosa
    Chronic severe depression
    Alcoholism
  Catabolic response
    Starvation
    Severe extensive burns

Table 8-6.   Some Potential Causes of Zinc Deficiency *(continued)*

Catabolic response (continued)
  Massive injury
  Chronic infectious disease
  Collagen vascular disease
  Recurrent severe fever
Parasitic disease
  Hookworm
  Schistosomiasis
  Giardiasis
  Malaria
Iatrogenic
  Antianabolic drugs
  Antimetabolite drugs
  Chelating drugs
  Diuretic drugs
  Severe surgical trauma
Pregnancy

keratotic dermatitis that usually begins around body orifices, failure to thrive, and impaired immune function. If untreated, the infants die. Recent studies suggest that a defect in tryptophan metabolism resulting in impaired synthesis of picolinic acid may be the cause of the impaired intestinal absorption of zinc in these infants (50, 159).

Very severe zinc deficiency may also occur in patients fed with parenteral alimentation fluids or oral formulas that are inadequate in zinc. The patients display low plasma zinc (160, 161), acrodermatitis (97, 162), impaired cell mediated immunity (96, 163), retarded healing, infection, and neuropsychological abnormalities (164). Utilization of amino acids and glucose is depressed (18). Factors contributing to the severity of the deficiency include increased loss of zinc associated with catabolism (86), intestinal malabsorption (165), liver disease (166), and the increased zinc requirement imposed by anabolism (18, 167). To prevent zinc deficiency in patients treated with total parenteral alimentation, the American Medical Association has recommended amounts of zinc for inclusion in parenteral fluids (168) (Table 8-7). These recommendations are conservative. They may be insufficient for patients who are experiencing massive fluid losses, or who have been very severely catabolic and are at present highly anabolic.

An important cause of conditioned zinc deficiency among free-living persons is alcoholic cirrhosis of the liver (166). Such individuals often

Table 8-7. Suggested Daily Intravenous Intake of Zinc (168)

	Pediatric Patients, μg/kg[a]	Stable Adult	Adult in Acute Catabolic State[b]	Stable Adult With Intestinal Losses[b]
Zinc	300[c] 100[d]	2.5−4.0 mg	Additional 2.0 mg	Add 12.2 mg/liter small-bowel fluid lost; 17.1 mg/kg of stool or ileos- tomy output[e]

[a]Limited data are available for infants weighing less than 1500 g. Their zinc requirement may be more than the recommendations because of their low body reserves and rapid growth.
[b]Frequent monitoring of blood levels in these patients is essential to provide proper dosage.
[c]Premature infants (weight less than 1500 g) up to 3 kg of body weight. Thereafter, the recommendations for full-term infants apply.
[d]Full-term infants and children up to 5 years of age. Thereafter the recommen- dations for adults apply, up to a maximum of 4 mg/day.
[e]Values derived by mathematical fitting of balance data from a 71-patient-week study in 24 patients (18).

have high urinary excretions of zinc when the liver injury is severe. Studies in rats suggest that substantial losses may also occur into the intestinal lumen (10). Abstinence from alcohol with recovery of liver function is often associated with improved zinc homeostasis. Patients with viral hepatitis may also have high excretions of zinc in urine (74). Other factors that contribute to the occurrence of zinc deficiency in such patients include low intakes of animal protein, intestinal malabsorption, and protein-losing enteropathy.

In addition to the signs of zinc deficiency noted previously in patients with iatrogenic zinc deficiency, patients with alcoholic liver disease have been found to have zinc-responsive night-blindness (10, 169). Testicular atrophy, impotence (169), poor healing, dysgeusia (10), disorientation, and hyperammonemia (170) in such patients may also be in part related to zinc depletion.

Zinc deficiency is a complication of intestinal malabsorption with or without inflammatory disease of the intestinal mucosa. Specific causes of deficiency include gluten enteropathy (171−174), Crohn's disease (18, 105, 151, 165, 175, 176), cystic fibrosis (177), giardiasis and stron- gyloidiasis associated with hypogammaglobulinemia (128, 178), and chronic pancreatitis. In addition to acrodermatitis (165) and other rashes such as dermatitis herpetiformis and chronic prurigo (173), the patients may display hypogeusia, growth failure, hypogonadism and infertility, poor healing, and impaired immunity.

Some patients with chronic renal disease become zinc deficient. The cause in most instances appears to be a low intake of readily available dietary zinc. Hemodialysis per se does not appear to cause zinc depletion (179). Signs of deficiency include depressed levels of plasma and hair zinc (180). Manifestations include hypogeusia (181) and impotence (182). Some patients with nephrotic syndrome display hyperzincuria (68, 75). The low levels of plasma and hair zinc in such patients probably are a reflection of dietary deficiency because the low plasma levels are out of proportion to the losses in urine and the binding of zinc to plasma albumin is substantially increased.

High erythrocyte turnover and excretion of the zinc from destroyed red blood cells is believed to be a factor in the zinc deficiency associated with hemolytic anemias such as thalassemia and sickle cell anemia (183–185). Low dietary zinc may be a contributing factor. Growth failure and hypogonadism occur in children and adolescents. Poor healing of leg ulcers occurs in patients with sickle cell disease (186). It is unclear whether other manifestations of sickle cell disease are improved by zinc therapy (187). A double-blind study study of 25 patients revealed a highly significant improvement in feeling of well-being, but no improvement in other symptoms or signs other than leg ulcer (188).

Patients with Down's syndrome may display signs of zinc deficiency including low plasma and leukocyte zinc (189) and zinc-responsive depressed immune functions (100). The mechanism for the impaired zinc homeostasis in such patients has not been identified.

Low plasma zinc consistent with zinc deficiency occurs in association with a variety of other conditions, such as chronic infection, cancer, and trauma (190). With catabolism, increased excretion of zinc occurs (86) and deficiency develops if intake is insufficient to compensate for these losses. As noted previously, anabolism without adequate zinc replacement exacerbates the deficiency.

Drugs may impair zinc homeostasis. For example, isoniazid inhibits the intestinal absorption of zinc (50), thiazides increase its excretion (70), and penicillamine increases its excretion and may cause clinical deficiency (191). Ethambutol, diasulfiram, oxyiquinolin, diodohydroxyquin, iproiazid, nialamide, isocarboxazid, and phentoin have all been implicated (192).

There is at present no evidence that impaired zinc nutriture contributes to the occurrence of diabetes mellitus. Some patients with diabetes mellitus may develop zinc deficiency because of poor dietary intake or because of other diseases which impair zinc metabolism. Increased urinary excretion of zinc appears to be partly responsible for growth failure and delayed sexual maturation in some children with diabetes mellitus (193).

The role of zinc in the taste acuity of humans has been a subject of controversy. In experimental animals (194) and humans (76), experimental zinc deficiency caused severe impairment of taste. In patients with alcoholic cirrhosis, hypogeusia may be caused either by zinc deficiency or by vitamin A deficiency (10). Several taste defects have been shown to be responsive to copper, zinc, or nickel (195). Thus zinc deficiency is not the only nutritional cause of impaired taste acuity. However, in a single-blind study, patients with idiopathic hypogeusia were found to respond to zinc (196). This was also true in a double-blind study of patients with uremia and hypogeusia (181). In contrast a double-blind study of patients with "idiopathic hypogeusia" was negative (197). A possible cause appears to have been a marked difference in the intestinal absorption of zinc among the subjects. A subgroup of "poor absorbers" responded to zinc and not to placebo while a second subgroup of "high absorbers" displayed improved taste following either zinc or the placebo (198). Perhaps the latter individuals absorbed zinc from their diets and thus recovered.

Zinc deprivation may have severe adverse effects on the eye. The cornea and retina contain about 460 $\mu g/Zn/g$ while the optic nerve contains about 120 $\mu g/Zn/g$ (192). Zinc is necessary for the function of retinol dehydrogenase (9), carbonic anhydrase, and lactic dehydrogenase of uveal and retinal tissue (192). As noted previously zinc-responsive impaired dark adaptation occurs in zinc-deficient patients with alcoholic liver disease (10). Optic neuritis and optic atrophy have also been attributed to zinc deficiency (191). A dyschromatopsia of the red–green color axis may occur and there may be irreversible injury of the retina (192).

EXPERIMENTAL ZINC DEFICIENCY IN HUMANS

Acute, severe zinc deficiency was produced in patients with scleroderma by oral administration of large amounts of histidine which caused massive zincurea (76). Signs of deficiency included tremor, ataxia, dysarthria, nystagmus, decreased vision, impaired thought processes, depression, euphoria, visual agnosia, receptive aphasia, dysgeusia, and dysomia. Recovery occurred soon after zinc supplementation.

Experimental dietary depletion in young women was produced by feeding a formula that provided less than 0.5 mg/day of zinc for 36 days. A substantial decline in plasma zinc occurred in 8 of 10 of the women (71, 72). Seven had nonspecific clinical abnormalities, including seborrheic dermatitis, staphylococcal cellulitis, sore throat, gingivitis, apthous stomatitis, headache, cracked nipples, diarrhea, and general malaise.

Less severe dietary depletion caused oligospermia in 4 of 5 men fed 2.7–5 mg/day of zinc for 24–44 weeks (199, 200). The decrease in sperm count coincided with a decrease in Leydig cell function. Plasma zinc, erythrocyte zinc, alkaline phosphatase, and lactic dehydrogenase decreased significantly, while levels of plasma ribonuclease and ammonia increased during depletion.

Zinc depletion in two young men fed about 3.8 mg of zinc daily for 16 weeks resulted in an initial decrease in urine and fecal zinc followed by a progressive increase in loss after about 8 weeks of depletion (94). Plasma zinc levels were similar at the beginning and end of depletion. Plasma cholesterol decreased about 20% and resting respiratory quotient decreased progressively even though the diet was rich in carbohydrate. Other changes included a decrease in plasma vitamin A and histidine, and surprisingly, an increase in serum alkaline phosphatase. Lymphocyte transformation in response to PHA and ConA was unchanged.

ZINC SUPPLEMENTATION AND THERAPY

The dosage of zinc given as therapy has varied widely in the past. This was in part because of a lack of knowledge of the most effective safe dose and the apparent wide range between nutritional requirements and evidence of toxicity in animals and man. Recent evidence suggests that tolerance may not be as great as previously thought. The administration of 160 mg of zinc to men for 5 weeks caused a 25% decrease in plasma HDL-cholesterol (201). Because of the role of HDL in transport of cholesterol from tissues to the liver for excretion, this effect of zinc may be deleterious. Other evidence of a need for caution is the finding in patients with sickle cell disease that pharmacologic amounts of zinc (150 mg daily) may interfere with the metabolism of copper sufficiently to impair hematopoiesis (202). Findings in sheep show that large amounts of zinc will cause abortion in that species (203). Presumably, humans may be similarly affected. These adverse effects of substantial doses of zinc suggest that caution may be appropriate in dispensing zinc to patients and others who wish to take a zinc "supplement." Until further evidence becomes available it seems prudent not to give more than 2–3 times the recommended dietary allowance of zinc to patients unless there is clear evidence of severe deficiency, excessive losses, or that intestinal absorption and retention are impaired.

Current data suggest that mild dietary zinc deficiency is not a rare phenomenon. The deficiency occurs in all population groups of both nonindustrial and industrial nations. Factors that contribute to its occurrence include limited availability of foods from which zinc is readily absorbed and a predominance of foods low in zinc or from which zinc is poorly absorbed. Conditioning factors often contribute to the occurrence of the deficiency. They include infections, parasitic diseases, intestinal malabsorption, severe liver disease, renal disease, severe catabolic responses, and certain inborn errors of metabolism. The major manifestations of zinc deficiencies include impaired growth and maturation, increased susceptibility to infection, poor healing, dermatitis, neuropsychological impairment, depressed vision, impaired taste and smell, and depressed gonadal function. There is at present no unequivocal diagnostic laboratory test of zinc deficiency. Proof of deficiency in some instances requires a controlled therapeutic intervention trial. Zinc supplementation should probably be limited to 2–3 times the recommended daily allowance unless there is a strong medical indication for a larger dose.

REFERENCES

1. W. R. Todd, C. A. Elvehjem, and E. B. Hart, *Am. J. Physiol.*, **107**, 146 (1934).
2. W. G. E. Eggleton, *Biochem. J.*, **34**, 991 (1940).
3. H. F. Tucker and W. D. Salmon, *Proc. Soc. Exp. Biol. Med.*, **88**, 613 (1955).
4. B. L. Vallee, W. E. C. Wacker, A. F. Bartholomay, and E. D. Robin, *N. Engl. J. Med.*, **255**, 403 (1956).
5. A. S. Prasad, A. Miale, Jr., Z. Farid, H. H. Sandstead, A. R. Schulert, and W. J. Darby, *Arch. Intern. Med.*, **111**, 407 (1963).
6. A. S. Prasad, A. Miale, Jr., Z. Farid, H. H. Sandstead, and A. R. Schulert, *J. Lab. Clin. Med.*, **61**, 537 (1963).
7. J. A. Halsted, H. A. Ronaghy, P. Abadi, M. Haghshenass, G. H. Amerhakemi, R. M. Barakat, and J. G. Reinhold, *Am. J. Med.*, **53**, 277 (1972).
8. J. F. Riordan, *Med. Clin. North Am.*, **60**, 661 (1976).
9. A. M. Huber and S. N. Gershoff, *J. Nutr.*, **105**, 1486 (1975).

10. R. M. Russel, *Am. J. Clin. Nutr.*, **33**, 2741 (1980).

11. A. S. Prasad, F. Fernandez-Madrid, and J. R. Ryan, *Am. J. Physiol.*, **236**, E272 (1979).

12. J. P. Slater, A. S. Midvan, and L. A. Loeb, *Biochem. Biophys. Res. Commun.*, **44**, 37 (1971).

13. D. S. Auld, H. Kawaguchi, D. M. Livingston, and B. L. Vallee, *Proc. Natl. Acad. Sci. USA*, **71**, 2091 (1974).

14. M. C. Scrutton, C. W. Wu, and D. A. Goldthwait, *Proc. Natl. Acad. Sci. USA*, **68**, 2497 (1971).

15. M. W. Terhune and H. H. Sandstead, *Science*, **177**, 68 (1972).

16. J. M. Hsu and R. L. Woosley, *J. Nutr.*, **102**, 1181 (1972).

17. J. A. Duerre, K. M. Ford, and H. H. Sandstead, *J. Nutr.*, **107**, 1082 (1977).

18. S. L. Wolman, G. H. Anderson, E. B. Marliss, and K. N. Jeejeebhoy, *Gastroenterology*, **76**, 458 (1979).

19. M. Kirchgessner, H. P. Roth, and E. Weigand, "Biochemical Changes in Zinc Deficiency," in A. S. Prasad, Ed., *Trace Elements in Human Health and Disease*, Part I, Academic Press, New York, 1976, p. 189.

20. M. Somers and E. J. Underwood, *Aust. J. Agr. Res.*, **20**, 899 (1969).

21. J. K. Chesters and J. Quarterman, *Br. J. Nutr.*, **24**, 1061 (1970).

22. E. Weigand and M. Kirchgessner, *J. Nutr.*, **110**, 469 (1980).

23. R. H. Follis, Jr., "Zinc," in *Deficiency Disease*, Charles C. Thomas, Springfield, Il., 1958, p. 69.

24. R. S. Pekarek, A. M. Hoagland, and M. C. Powanda, *Nutr. Rep. Int.*, **16**, 267 (1977).

25. R. W. Luecke, E. Charles, C. E. Simonel, and P. J. Fraker, *J. Nutr.*, **108**, 881 (1978).

26. P. J. Fraker, P. DePasquale-Jardieu, C. M. Zwickl, and R. W. Luecke, *Proc. Natl. Acad. Sci. USA*, **75**, 5660 (1978).

27. H. H. Sandstead, V. C. Lanier, Jr., G. H. Shepard, and D. D. Gillespie, *Am. J. Clin. Nutr.*, **23**, 514 (1970).

28. J. Apgar, *J. Nutr.*, **100**, 470 (1970).

29. H. Swenerton and L. S. Hurley, *J. Nutr.*, **110**, 575 (1980).

30. G. H. Barney, M. C. Orgebin-Crist, and M. P. Macapinlac, *J. Nutr.*, **95**, 526 (1968).

31. L. S. Hurley and H. Swenerton, *Proc. Soc. Exp. Biol. Med.*, **123**, 692 (1966).

32. J. Apgar, *J. Nutr.*, **102**, 343 (1972).

33. S. J. Buell, G. J. Fosmire, D. A. Ollerich, and H. H. Sandstead, *Exp. Neurol.*, **55**, 199 (1977).

34. J. M. McKenzie, G. J. Fosmire, and H. H. Sandstead, *J. Nutr.*, **105**, 1466 (1975).

35. C. Dvergsten and H. Sandstead, *Fed. Proc.*, **39**, 431 (1980).

36. P. M. Lokken, E. S. Halas, and H. H. Sandstead, *Proc. Soc. Exp. Biol. Med.*, **144**, 680 (1973).

37. E. S. Halas, M. C. Rowe, O. R. Johnson, J. M. McKenzie, and H. H. Sandstead, "Effects of Intra-Uterine Zinc Deficiency on Subsequent Behavior," in A. S. Prasad, Ed., *Trace Elements in Human Health and Disease*, Part I, Academic Press, New York, 1976, p. 327.

38. E. S. Halas, G. M. Reynolds, and H. H. Sandstead, *Physiol. Behav.*, **19**, 653 (1977).

39. E. S. Halas, P. A. Burger, and H. H. Sandstead, *Fed. Proc.*, **37**, 889 (1978).

40. E. S. Halas, M. D. Heinrich, and H. H. Sandstead, *Physiol. Behav.*, **22**, 991 (1979).

41. H. H. Sandstead, D. A. Strobel, G. M. Logan, Jr., E. O. Marks, and R. A. Jacob, *Am. J. Clin. Nutr.*, **31**, 844 (1978).

42. D. Strobel, H. Sandstead, L. Zimmerman, and A. Reuter, "Prenatal Protein and Zinc Malnutrition," in G. Rupenthal, Ed., *Advances in Primatology, Nursery Care of Non-Human Primates*, Plenum, New York, 1980, p. 43.

43. G. W. Hesse, *Science*, **205**, 1005 (1979).

44. J. Wallwork and H. H. Sandstead, *Fed. Proc.*, **40**, 939 (1981).

45. D. L. Antonson, A. J. Barak, and J. A. VanderLoof, *J. Nutr.*, **109**, 142 (1980).

46. A. H. Methfessel and H. Spencer, *J. Appl. Physiol.*, **34**, 58 (1973).

47. N. T. Davies, *Br. J. Nutr.*, **43**, 189 (1980).

48. H. Spencer, B. Rosoff, I. Lewin, and J. Samachson, "Studies of Zinc-65 Metabolism in Man," in A. S. Prasad, Ed., *Zinc Metabolism*, Charles C. Thomas, Springfield, Il., 1966, p. 339.

49. M. K. Song and N. F. Adham, *J. Nutr.*, **109**, 2152 (1980).

50. G. W. Evans, *Nutr. Rev.*, **38**, 137 (1980).

51. R. J. Cousins, *Nutr. Rev.*, **37**, 97 (1979).

52. K. T. Smith and R. J. Cousins, *J. Nutr.*, **110**, 316 (1980).

53. B. C. Starcher, J. G. Glauber, and J. G. Madaras, *J. Nutr.*, **110**, 1391 (1980).

54. G. W. Evans, *Proc. Soc. Exp. Biol. Med.*, **151**, 775 (1976).

55. D. Van Campen and W. A. House, *J. Nutr.*, **104**, 84 (1974).

56. B. Sandström, B. Arvidsson, A. Cederblad, and E. Björn-Rasmussen, *Am. J. Clin. Nutr.*, **33**, 739 (1980).

57. J. M. McKenzie and N. T. Davies, personal communication (1980).

58. G. W. Evans and E. C. Johnson, *J. Nutr.*, **110**, 1076 (1980).

59. N. T. Davies and R. Nightingale, *Br. J. Nutr.*, **34**, 243 (1975).

60. C. Kies, H. M. Fox, and B. Beshgetoor, *Cereal Chem.*, **56**, 133 (1979).

61. F. Ismail-Beigi, B. Faraji, and J. G. Reinhold. *Am. J. Clin. Nutr.*, **30**, 1721 (1977).

62. J. W. Erdman, K. E. Weingartner, G. C. Mustakas, R. D. Schmutz, H. M. Parker, and R. M. Forbes, *J. Food Sci.*, **45**, 1193 (1980).

63. A. L. Camire and F. M. Clydesdale, *J. Food Sci.*, in press.

64. J. L. Kelsay, R. A. Jacob, and E. S. Prather, *Am. J. Clin. Nutr.*, **32**, 2307 (1979).

65. N. W. Solomons, R. A. Jacob, O. Pineda, and F. E. Viteri, *J. Lab. Clin. Med.*, **94**, 335 (1979).

66. N. W. Solomons, R. A. Jacob, O. Pineda, and F. E. Viteri, *J. Nutr.*, **109**, 1519 (1979).

67. J. A. Halsted, J. C. Smith, Jr., and M. I. Irwin, *J. Nutr.*, **104**, 345 (1974).

68. R. A. McCance and E. M. Widdowson, *Biochem. J.*, **36**, 692 (1942).

69. P. E. Stake, W. J. Miller, D. M. Blackmon, R. P. Gentry, and M. W. Neathery, *J. Nutr.*, **104**, 1279 (1974).

70. R. I. Henkin, "Zinc in Humans," in R.I. Henkin and Committee, Eds., *Zinc*, University Park Press, Baltimore, 1979, p. 123.

71. F. M. Hess, J. C. King, and S. Margen, *J. Nutr.*, **107**, 1610 (1977).

72. F. M. Hess, J. C. King, and S. Margen, *J. Nutr.*, **107**, 2219 (1977).

73. J. F. Sullivan, *Gastroenterology*, **42**, 439 (1962).

74. R. I. Henkin and F. R. Smith, *Am. J. Med. Sci.*, **264**, 401 (1972).

75. E. W. Reimold, *Am. J. Dis. Child.*, **134** 46 (1980).

76. R. I. Henkin, B. Patten, P. Re, and D. A. Bonzert, *Arch. Neurol.*, **32**, 745 (1975).

77. J. B. Freeman, L. D. Stegink, P. D. Meyer, L. K. Fry, and L. Denbesten, *J. Surg. Res.*, **18**, 463 (1975).

78. R. A. Jacob, H. H. Sandstead, J. M. Munoz, L. M. Klevay, and D. B. Milne, *Am. J. Clin. Nutr.*, in press.

79. A. S. Prasad, A. R. Schulert, H. H. Sandstead, A. Miale, Jr., and Z. Farid, *J. Lab. Clin. Med.*, **62**, 84 (1963).

80. E. L. Giroux, M. Durieux, and P. J. Schechter, *Bioinorg. Chem.*, **5**, 211 (1976).

81. M. D. Lifschitz and R. I. Henkin, *J. Appl. Physiol.*, **31**, 88 (1971).

82. J. D. Bogden, "Blood Zinc in Health and Disease," in J.O. Nriagu, Ed., *Zinc in the Environment: Healthy Sex*, Part 2, Wiley, New York, 1980, p. 137.

83. A. S. Prasad, "Zinc in Human Nutrition," in *CRC Critical Review in Clinical Laboratory Science*, Chemical Rubber Co., Cleveland, 1977, p. 1.

84. R. L. Aamodt, W. F. Rumble, G. S. Johnston, D. Foster, and R. I. Henkin, *Am. J. Clin. Nutr.*, **32**, 559 (1979).

85. K. H. Falchuk, *N. Engl. J. Med.*, **296**, 1129 (1977).

86. W. R. Beisel, R. S. Pekarek, and R. W. Wannemacher, Jr., "Homeostatic Mechanisms Affecting Plasma Zinc Levels in Acute Stress," in A.S. Prasad, Ed., *Trace Elements in Human Health and Disease*, Vol. I, Academic, New York, 1976, p. 87.

87. I. Bremner and N. T. Davies, *Biochem. J.*, **149**, 733 (1975).

88. S. H. Oh and P. D. Whanger, *Am. J. Physiol.*, **237**, E18 (1979).

89. J. F. Ross, F. G. Ebaugh, Jr., and T. R. Talbot, Jr., *Trans. Assoc. Am. Physicians*, **71**, 322 (1958).

90. L. S. Hurley and S. Tau, *Am. J. Physiol.*, **222**, 322 (1972).

91. E. C. Savlov, W. H. Strain, and F. Huegin, *J. Surg. Res.*, **2**, 209 (1962).

92. E. L. Lichti, J. A. Schilling, and H. M. Shurley, *Am. J. Surg.*, **123**, 253 (1972).

93. N. W. Solomons, *Am. J. Clin. Nutr.*, **32**, 856 (1979).

94. H. Sandstead, L. Klevay, J. Mahalko, L. Inman, W. Bolonchuk, H. Lukaski, G. Lykken, T. Kramer, L. Johnson, D. Milne, and J. Wallwork, *Clin. Res.*, **28**, 600A (1980).

95. K. M. Hambidge, C. Hambidge, M. Jacobs, and J. D. Baum, *Pediatr. Res.*, **6**, 868 (1972).

96. R. S. Pekarek, H. H. Sandstead, R. A. Jacob, and D. F. Barcome, *Am. J. Clin. Nutr.*, **32**, 1466 (1979).

97. T. Arakawa, T. Tamura, Y. Igarashi, H. Suzuki, and H. H. Sandstead, *Am. J. Clin. Nutr.*, **29**, 197 (1976).

98. M. H. Golden, A. A. Jackson, and B. E. Golden, *Lancet*, **2**, 1057 (1977).

99. M. H. N. Golden, B. E. Golden, P. S. E. G. Harland, and A. A. Jackson, *Lancet*, **1**, 1226 (1978).

100. B. Björrksten, O. Beck, K. H. Gustavson, G. Hallmann, B. Hägglof, and T. Tärnvik, *Acta Paediatr. Scand.*, **69**, 183 (1980).

101. P. R. Gordon and B. L. O'Dell, *J. Nutr.*, **110**, 2125 (1980).

102. E. W. Murphy, B. W. Willis, and B. K. Watts, *J. Am. Diet. Assoc.*, **6**, 345 (1975).

103. National Research Council, *The Contribution of Drinking Water to Mineral Nutrition of Humans*, National Academy of Science, Washington, D.C., 1979.

104. A. Pecoud, P. Donzel, and J. L. Schelling, *Clin. Pharmacol. Ther.*, **17**, 469 (1975).

105. H. H. Sandstead, *Am. J. Clin. Nutr.*, **26**, 1251 (1973).

106. H. H. Sandstead, L. M. Klevay, R. A. Jacob, J. M. Munoz, G. M. Logan, Jr., S. J. Reck, F. R. Dintzis, G. E. Inglett, and W. C. Shuey, "Effects of Dietary Fiber and Protein Level on Mineral Element Metabolism," in G.E. Inglett, Ed., *Dietary Fibers: Chemistry and Nutrition*, Academic, New York, 1979, p. 147.

107. World Health Organization, "Zinc," in *Trace Elements in Human Nutrition*, Technical Report #532, Geneva, 1973, p. 9.

108. National Research Council, "Zinc," in *Recommended Dietary Allowances*, 9th Revised Edition, National Academy of Science, Washington, D.C., 1980.

109. E. M. Widdowson, "Chemical Analysis of the Body," in J. Brozek, Ed., *Human Body Composition*, Pergamon, Oxford, 1965, p. 31.

110. G. B. Forbes and J. B. Hirsch, *Ann. N.Y. Acad. Sci.*, **110**, 255 (1963).

111. E. J. Underwood, "Zinc," in *Trace Elements in Human and Animal Nutrition*, 4th ed., Academic, New York, 1976, p. 196.

112. J. D. Fomon, *Infant Nutrition*, Saunders, Philadelphia, 1967, p. 30.

113. P. A. Walravens and K. M. Hambidge, *Am. J. Clin. Nutr.*, **29**, 1114 (1976).

114. K. W. Hambidge, P. A. Walravens, C. E. Casey, R. M. Brown, and C. Bender, *J. Pediatr.*, **94**, 607 (1979).

115. G. W. Evans and P. E. Johnson, *Pediatr. Res.*, **14**, 876 (1980).

116. L. S. Hurley, B. Lönnerdal, and A. G. Stanislowski, *Lancet*, **1**, 677 (1979).

117. M. J. Dauncey, J. C. L. Shaw, and J. Urman, *Pediatr. Res.*, **11**, 991 (1977).

118. J. C. L. Shaw, *Am. J. Dis. Child.*, **133**, 1260 (1979).

119. R. Berfenstam, *Acta Pediatr.*, **41** (suppl. 87), 1 (1952).

120. B. Momćilovic, B. Belonge, A. Giroux, and B. G. Shaw, *J. Nutr.*, **106**, 913 (1976).

121. S. J. Ritchey, M. K. Korslund, L. M. Gilbert, D. C. Fay, and M. R. Robinson, *Am. J. Clin. Nutr.*, **32**, 799 (1979).

122. J. L. Greger, S. C. Zaikis, R. P. Abernathy, O. A. Bennett, and J. Juffman, *J. Nutr.*, **108**, 1449 (1978).

123. A. S. Prasad, H. H. Sandstead, A. R. Schulert, and A. S. El Rooby, *J. Lab. Clin. Med.*, **62**, 591 (1963).

124 H. H. Sandstead, A. S. Prasad, A. R. Schulert, Z. Farid, A. Miale, Jr., S. Bassilly, and W. J. Darby, *Am. J. Clin. Nutr.*, **20**, 422 (1967).

125. A. S. Prasad, J. A. Halsted, and M. Nadimi, *Am. J. Med.*, **31**, 532 (1961).

126. Y. D. Coble, Jr., C. W. Bardin, G. T. Ross, and W. J. Darby, *J. Clin. Endocrinol.*, **32**, 361 (1971).

127. A. Arcásoy, A. O. Cavdar, and E. Babacan, *Acta Haemat.*, **60**, 76 (1978).

128. J. Caggiano, R. Schnitzler, W. Strauss, R. K. Baker, A. C. Carter, A. S. Josephson, and S. Wallach, *Am. J. Med., Sci.*, **257**, 305 (1969).

129. C. Chao-ling, C. Shih-Tao, C. Kuo-Chien, Y. Lan-Sheng, L. Sheng-Ch'ing, L. Chih-Sen, K. Ch'ing-Yun, L. Yu-Fed, and H. Ching-Ya, *Chinese Med. J.*, **79**, 26 (1959).

130. I. I. Lemann, *Arch. Int. Med.,* **16,** 139 (1910).

131. H. H. Sandstead, A. S. Shukry, A. S. Prasad, M. K. Gabr, A. El-Hefney, N. Mokhtar, and W. J. Darby, *Am. J. Clin. Nutr.,* **17,** 15 (1965).

132. H. A. Ronaghy, J. G. Reinhold, M. Mahloudji, P. Ghavami, M. R. S. Fox, and J. A. Halsted, *Am. J. Clin. Nutr.,* **27,** 112 (1974).

133. A. S. Prasad, A. R. Schulert, A. Miale, Jr., Z. Farid, and H. H. Sandstead, *Am. J. Clin. Nutr.,* **12,** 437 (1963).

134. Y. D. Coble, A. R. Schulert, and Z. Farid, *Am. J. Clin. Nutr.,* **18,** 421 (1966).

135. A. O. Çavdar, E. Babacon, A. Arcásoy, and U. Ertem, *Am. J. Clin. Nutr.,* **33,** 542 (1980).

136. L. S. Hurley, J. Gowan, and H. Swenerton, *Teratology,* **4,** 199 (1971).

137. L. S. Hurley and R. E. Shrader, *Nature,* **254,** 427 (1975).

138. L. E. Sever and I. Emanuel, *Teratology,* **7,** 117 (1973).

139. D. J. Verburg, L. I. Burd, E. O. Hoxtell, and L. K. Merrill, *Obstet. Gynecol.,* **44,** 233 (1974).

140. K. M. Hambidge, K. H. Neldner, and P. A. Walravens, *Lancet,* **1,** 77 (1975).

141. G. P. Butrimovitz and W. C. Purdy, "Plasma Zinc Concentrations Throughout Childhood," in S. Meites, Ed., *Pediatric Clinical Chemistry. A Survey of Normals, Methods and Instrumentation, With Commentary,* American Association for Clinical Chemists, Washington, D.C., 1977, p. 230.

142. G. P. Butrimovitz and W. C. Purdy, *Am. J. Clin. Nutr.,* **31,** 1409 (1978).

143. K. M. Hambidge, P. A. Walravens, S. White, M. L. Anthony, and M. L. Roth, *Am. J. Clin. Nutr.,* **29,** 734 (1976).

144. H. A. White, *J. Am. Diet. Assoc.,* **68,** 243 (1976).

145. G. Michaëlsson, L. Juhlin, and A. Valquist, *Arch. Dermatol.,* **113,** 31 (1976).

146. G. Michaëlsson, L. Juhlin, and L. Ljunghall, *Br. J. Dermatol.,* **97,** 561 (1977).

147. G. Michaëlsson, A. Valquist, and L. Juhlin, *Br. J. Dermatol.,* **96,** 283 (1977).

148. K. M. Hambidge and W. Droegmueller, *Obstet. Gynecol.,* **44,** 666 (1974).

149. R. Giroux, P. J. Schechter, and J. Schoun, *Clin. Sci. Mol. Med.,* **51,** 545 (1976).

150. W. Crosby, J. Metcoff, P. Costello, M. Mameesh, H. Sandstead, R. Jacob, P. McClain, G. Jacobson, W. Reid, and G. Burns, *J. Obstet. Gynecol.,* **128,** 22 (1977).

151. S. Jameson, *Acta Med. Scand.* (Supple. 593), 4 (1976).

152. J. Metcoff, P. Costiloe, W. Crosby, S. Dutta, H. Sandstead, and C. E. Bodwell, *Am. J. Clin. Nutr.,* in press.

153. J. L. Greger, *J. Geront.,* **32,** 549 (1977).

154. J. L. Greger and B. S. Sciscoe, *J. Am. Diet. Assoc.,* **70,** 37 (1977).

155. P. A. Wagner, M. L. Krista, L. B. Bailey, G. J. Christakis, J. A. Jernigan, P. E. Aravjo, H. Appledorf, C. G. Davis, and J. S. Dinning, *Am. J. Clin. Nutr.,* **33,** 1771 (1980).

156. T. Hällbook and E. Lanner, *Lancet,* **2,** 780 (1972).

157. K. Haeger and E. Lanner, *J. Vas. Dis.,* **3,** 77 (1974).

158. K. M. Hambidge, K. H. Neldner, P. A. Walravens, W. L. Weston, A. Silverman, J. L. Sabol, and R. M. Brown, "Zinc and Acrodermatitis Enteropathica," in K. M. Hambidge and B. L. Nichols, Eds., *Zinc and Copper in Clinical Medicine,* Spectrum, New York, 1978, p. 81.

159. I. Krieger, *Nutr. Rev.*, **38**, 148 (1980).

160. N. W. Solomons, T. J. Layden, I. H. Rosenberg, K. Vo-Khactu, and H. H. Sandstead, *Gastroenterology*, **70**, 1022 (1976).

161. C. R. Fleming, R. E. Hodges, and L. S. Hurley, *Am. J. Clin. Nutr.*, **29**, 70 (1976).

162. R. G. Kay, C. Tasman-Jones, J. Pybus, R. Whiting, and H. Block, *Ann. Surg.*, **183**, 331 (1976).

163. J. M. Oleske, M. L. Westphal, S. Shore, D. Gorden, J. D. Bogden, and A. Nahmis, *Am. J. Dis. Child.*, **133**, 915 (1979).

164. C. Tasman-Jones, R. G. Kay, and S. P. Lee, *Surg. Ann.*, **10**, 23 (1978).

165. C. McClain, C. Soutor, and L. Zieve, *Gastroenterology*, **78**, 272 (1980).

166. J. F. Sullivan and R. E. Burch, "Potential Role of Zinc in Liver Disease," in A.S. Prasad, Ed., *Trace Elements in Human Health and Disease*, Part I, Academic, New York, 1976, p. 67.

167. J. Latimer, C. McClain, and H. Sharp, *J. Pediatr.*, **97**, 434 (1980).

168. American Medical Association, *J.A.M.A.*, **241**, 2051 (1979).

169. C. J. McClain, D. H. Van Thiel, S. Parker, L. K. Badzin, and H. Gilbert, *Alcoholism: Clin. Exp. Res.*, **3**, 135 (1979).

170. P. Rabbani and A. S. Prasad, *Am. J. Physiol.*, **235**, E203 (1978).

171. N. W. Solomons, I. H. Rosenberg, and H. H. Sandstead, *Am. J. Clin. Nutr.*, **29**, 371 (1976).

172. A. H. G. Love, M. Elmes, M. K. Golden, and D. McMaster, "Zinc Deficiency and Coeliac Disease," in M. McNicholl, C. F. McCarthy, and P. F. Fottrell, Eds., *Perspectives in Coeliac Disease*, University Park Press, Baltimore, 1978, p. 335.

173. F. Bauer, *Aust. J. Derm.*, **19**, 104 (1978).

174. P. E. Jones, C. Seldon, and T. J. Peters, *Gut*, **20**, A922 (1979).

175. P. Merianos, *Br. J. Med.*, **1**, 316 (1975).

176. N. W. Solomons, I. H. Rosenberg, H. H. Sandstead, and K. P. Khactu, *Digestion*, **16**, 87 (1977).

177. R. A. Jacob, H. H. Sandstead, N. W. Solomons, R. Rieger, and R. Rothberg, *Am. J. Clin. Nutr.*, **31**, 638 (1978).

178. H. H. Sandstead, personal observation.

179. Th. Mountokalakis, D. Dakanalis, D. Boukis, K. Virvidakis, S. Voudiklari, and A. Koutselinis, *Clin. Nephrol.*, **12**, 206 (1979).

180. S. K. Mahajan, A. S. Prasad, P. Rabbani, W. A. Briggs, and F. McDonald, *J. Lab. Clin. Med.*, **94**, 693 (1979).

181. J. C. Burge, H. S. Park, C. P. Whitlock, and R. A. Schemmel, *Kidney Int.*, **15**, 49 (1979).

182. L. D. Antoniou, R. L. Shalhoub, T. Sudhaker, and J. C. Smith, Jr., *Lancet*, **2**, 895 (1977).

183. A. S. Prasad, M. Diwany, M. Gabr, H. H. Sandstead, N. Mokhtar, and A. El Hefney, *Ann. Intern. Med.*, **62**, 87 (1965).

184. A. S. Prasad, E. B. Schoomaker, J. Ortega, G. J. Brewer, D. Oberleas, and F. J. Oelshlegel, *Clin. Chem.*, **21**, 582 (1975).

185. U. Doğru, A. Arcásoy, and A. O. Çavdar, *Acta Haemat.*, **62**, 41 (1979).

186. G. R. Serjeant, R. E. Galloway, and M. C. Gueri, *Lancet*, **2**, 819 (1970).

187. A. S. Prasad, "Role of Zinc in Humans," in *Ultratrace Metal Analysis in Science and Environment*, American Chemical Society, 1979, p. 197.

188. M. Koshy, H. H. Sanstead, R. A. Jacob, L. Williams, and G. Logan, "Zinc Supplementation in Sickle Cell Anemia," in *Mutant Hemoglobins*, University of Chicago Press, 1981.

189. A. Milunsky, B. M. Hackley, and J. A. Halsted, *J. Ment. Defic. Res.*, **14**, 99 (1970).

190. H. H. Sandstead, K. P. Vo-Khactu, and N. Solomons, "Conditioned Zinc Deficiency," in A.S. Prasad, Ed., *Trace Elements in Human Health and Disease*, Part I, Academic, New York, 1976, p. 33.

191. W. G. Klingberg, A. S. Prasad, and D. Oberleas, "Zinc Deficiency Following Pencillamine Therapy," in A.S. Prasad, Ed., *Trace Elements in Human Health and Disease*, Part I, Academic, New York, 1976, p. 51.

192. I. H. Leopold, *Am. J. Ophthalmol.*, **85**, 871 (1978).

193. W. Canfield, personal communication, 1981.

194. F. A. Catalanotta, *J. Nutr.*, **109**, 1079 (1979).

195. R. I. Henkin, P. P. G. Graziadei, and D. F. Bradley, *Ann. Int. Med.*, **71**, 791 (1969).

196. P. J. Schecter, W. T. Friedewald, D. A. Bonzert, M. S. Raff, and R. I. Henkin, "Ideopathic Hypogeusia: A Description of the Syndrome and a Single Blind Study with Zinc Sulfate," in C. Pfeiffer, Ed., *International Review of Neurobiology*, Suppl 1, Academic, New York, 1972, p. 125.

197. R. I. Henkin, P. J. Schecter, W. T. Friedwald, D. L. Demits, and M. Raff., *Am. J. Med. Sci.*, **272**, 285 (1976).

198. R. I. Henkin, personal communication, 1980.

199. A. S. Prasad, P. Rabbani, A. Abbasi, E. Bowersox, and M. R. S. Fox, *Ann. Int. Med.*, **89** 483 (1978).

200. A. A. Abbasi, A. S. Prasad, P. Rabbani, and E. DuMouchelle, *J. Lab. Clin. Med.*, **96**, 544 (1980).

201. P. L. Hooper, L. Visconti, P. J. Garry, and G. E. Johnson, *J.A.M.A.*, **244**, 1960 (1980).

202. A. S. Prasad, G. J. Brewer, E. B. Schoomaker, and P. Rabbani, *J.A.M.A.*, **240**, 2166 (1978).

203. J. K. Campbell and C. F. Mills, *Environ, Res.*, **20**, 1 (1979).

PART 4

Nutrition in Diseases Common in Adolescence

9

Keshan Disease and Selenium in China

KESHAN DISEASE RESEARCH GROUP OF CHINESE
ACADEMY OF MEDICAL SCIENCES, KEYOU GE, M.D.,
PRESENTING

Institute of Health, Beijing, China

THE RECOGNITION OF KESHAN DISEASE

Keshan disease is an endemic cardiomyopathy of unknown cause. Since 1935 when this disease was recognized in Keshan, a county located in northeast China, more and more areas have been found affected. The affected areas, most of them separated from each other, are located in a long beltlike zone running across the country from northeast to southwest. Between affected and nonaffected areas, an intermediate zone with gradually decreasing incidence rate could be demonstrated in some districts.

The disease occurs most frequently in rural areas and predominantly in peasants. The most susceptible groups are children below 10 years old and women of childbearing age. More than 10 million people are living in affected areas.

Keshan disease had been divided into several clinicopathological types: acute, subacute, chronic, and latent. The acute type occurs suddenly and death may occur from cardiogenic shock in a few hours. Chronic cases may persist a number of years with varying degrees of congestive heart failure. The subacute type, most commonly seen in children, has clinical manifestations that are intermediate between the acute and chronic types. The mortality was rather high. Half of the acute and subacute cases died in three to four subsequent years of our observation.

The principal pathological change of Keshan disease is multifocal necrosis of myocardium. The heart usually appears more or less ball-shaped with the dilatation of all chambers. Necrotic foci of various size and various stages of organization are disseminated throughout the myocardium and they are often joined to each other representing a networklike lesion in the ventricular wall. Electron microscopy revealed that the most common and conspicuous change was found in mitochondria. Myocytolysis, the fundamental pathological change of most cases, appears to be started with mitochondrial disorganization. Myofibrillar atrophy and fragmentation occur consequently and finally result in complete destruction of the cardiocytes (1). Changes in other organs are usually not appreciable.

THE SELENIUM STATUS OF INHABITANTS

Since white muscle disease, a known selenium-deficiency disease in animals, was found to be prevalent in some places located in the same belt and the manifestations as well as the pathological changes of involved cattle somewhat resemble those of Keshan disease, the selenium status of inhabitants was studied in connection with the prevalence of Keshan disease (2).

About 5000 samples of human hair and staple grains were collected from 71 affected sites in 47 counties within the long belt and from 125 nonaffected sites in 77 counties within or far from the belt. The geographical features of these sampling sites include hilly and mountainous regions, plains and coastal areas, salted and nonsalted soils, and so forth. All the samples collected were analyzed by a fluorometric method for their selenium content (3).

The analytical data indicate that the inhabitants living in affected areas are exclusively selenium deficient. The average selenium content of 1478 hair samples collected from affected areas was 0.074 ppm and that of 1614 samples from nonaffected areas was 0.343 ppm. If each sampling site is taken as a unit, the hair selenium levels of the population living in affected sites were all below 0.12 ppm, whereas in nonaffected sites they were all about 0.20 ppm. People who live in the intermediate zone between affected and nonaffected areas have a level of 0.12−0.20 ppm. In northwestern and southeastern districts far from the long belt, the hair selenium contents are much higher than in the nonaffected sites located within the belt, going up to 0.25−0.60 ppm.

Table 9-1.   Whole Blood GSH-px Activities ($X \pm$ SE) of Affected and Nonaffected Area Inhabitants

Areas	Number of Subjects	Average GSH-px Activity, unit[a]
Outskirts of Beijing (nonaffected)	22	77.5 ± 2.1
Outskirts of Chengdu (nonaffected)	20	73.6 ± 3.1
Mianing county, Sichuan (affected)	63	60.5 ± 0.7
Zhouxizn county, Shandang (affected)	20	61.9 ± 2.8

[a]Decreasing in number of μM of GSH after incubation in five minutes with 8 μl of whole blood and from which the nonenzymic value has been subtracted.

The whole blood glutathione peroxidase activity was measured by Halfman's method (4). The estimation showed the same accuracy in the susceptible population as in controls (Table 9-1). The average enzyme activity of people in affected areas is significantly lower than that of people in nonaffected areas.

A selenium loading test was also carried out for evaluation of selenium status. Children of 5 to 7 years old from both affected and nonaffected areas were given a loading dose of 250 μg of selenium (as aqueous solution of sodium selenite) after dinner. Twelve-hour night urine samples were collected and analyzed. The result confirmed again that the affected children were selenium deficient. They excreted only 1.7% of the loading dosage, more after loading than before (Table 9-2).

The inhabitants of rural areas rely essentially on local foods. The low selenium content of grains produced in endemic areas should be the

Table 9-2.   Quantity[a] of Se excreted in Urine of Affected and Nonaffected Area Inhabitants Before and After an Oral Dosage of 250 μg Se (as Na_2SeO_3)

Population	Number of Subjects	Before Loading (μg)	After Loading (μg)	Difference Value (μg)	As Percentage of Loading Dosage
Affected area with Se supplementa-tion	7	2.16 ±0.28	12.99 ±2.83	10.82 ±2.58	4.3 ±0.71
Nonaffected areas	10	1.50 ±0.04	8.4 ±3.16	6.9 ±1.21	2.7 ±0.56
Affected areas	9	0.69 ±0.06	4.92 ±1.24	4.23 ±1.26	1.7 ±0.50

[a]$X \pm$ SE.

explanation of the selenium-deficient status of the affected population. Wheat, corn, rice, and soybeans raised in affected areas contain only 1/8 to 1/4 the amount of selenium of the same kinds of grains raised in nonaffected areas (Table 9-3). In addition, some selected sites were studied in contrast with proper controls (Table 9-4). In all pairs of affected and nonaffected sites, the selenium contents of grains fit the rule mentioned above and also associated well with the hair selenium levels of the local people.

THE EFFECT OF SODIUM SELENITE ON THE PREVENTION OF KESHAN DISEASE

There had been no effective method of prevention since Keshan disease was first recognized. Based on the studies of lack of toxicity of sodium selenite and the encouraging results of limited human trials, the preventive effect of sodium selenite was tested in 1974–1977 in Mianing county, Sichuan province (5). All children 1–9 years old in 119 production teams of three people's communes were observed in 1974, and the group was expanded to 169 teams of four communes in 1975. Half of the children were given sodium selenite tablets once a week and the other half placebo. The dosage was as follows: 1–5 years, 0.5 mg, 6–9 years, 1.0 mg of sodium selenite. The treated and control groups were randomly selected and were not changed during the 2 years of observation.

A Keshan Disease Hospital was established in the area under investi-

Table 9-3. Selenium Content of Grains of Different Areas

Areas	Corn $\overline{X}\pm SE$	Wheat $\overline{X}\pm SE$	Rice $\overline{X}\pm SE$	Soybean $\overline{X}\pm SE$
Affected	0.0045 ±0.0002 (178)[a]	0.0079 ±0.0006 (116)	0.0069 ±0.0004 (49)	0.0098 ±0.0007 (134)
Nonaffected	0.0355 ±0.0062 (82)	0.0315 ±0.0004 (30)	0.0239 ±0.0054 (49)	0.0689 ±0.0139 (30)

[a]In parentheses are number of samples.

Table 9-4. Regional Characteristics of Keshan Disease Prevalence and the Selenium Level of the Areas (ppm)

Areas	Hair	Soybean	Rice	Wheat	Sweet Potato	Oat
Hilly region (affected)	0.097–0.123 (79)[a]	0.020–0.034 (9)			0.0029–0.0046 (15)	
Coastal region (nonaffected)	0.234–0.331 (40)	0.042–0.074 (4)			0.075–0.089 (4)	
Mountainous (affected)	0.084 (20)	0.020 (3)				
Plain (nonaffected)	0.204–0.228 (40)	0.041–0.081 (4)				
Nonsalted (affected)	0.056 (20)			0.0053 (6)		0.0053 (5)
Salted soil (nonaffected)	0.170 (20)			0.0196 (6)		0.0395 (4)
Surrounding (affected)	0.060 (18)	0.0057 (4)	0.0078 (5)			
Safety island (nonaffected)	0.114 (20)	0.025 (5)	0.0202 (6)			

[a]In parentheses are the number of samples.

gation. Diagnoses of the disease were done according to the Clinical Diagnostic Criteria drawn up by the National Conference of the Etiology of Keshan Disease in 1974. Patients were reexamined each year until 1977. Only the acute and subacute cases were included in the mortality statistics.

The incidence rate is shown in Table 9-5. In control groups, there were 54 and 42 new cases out of 3985 and 5445 subjects in 1974 and 1975. The incidence rate was 13.5 and 9.5 per 1000. In the selenium treated group, however, there were only 10 and 7 cases, respectively. The incidence rate was 2.2 and 1.0 per 1000. The difference between the two groups was statistically significant ($p < 0.01$).

Since the preventive effects were significant in the first two test years, all children were given selenium in the subsequent years. A control group was omitted. In 1976, only 4 cases occurred out of 12,579 treated children, the incidence rate being 0.32/1000. In 1977, none was found among 12,744 subjects. There were 4 cases in observed communes; however, all of them were above 10 years old, outside the limits of the observation.

The results also indicate a better prognosis of patients in the treated group than that in the placebo group. By the end of 1977, 53 cases of the 106 in control groups died. The case fatality rate was 50%. In the selenium treated group, however, there was only one death. The case fatality rate was as low as 6%. In addition, 12 of the 51 survivors in control groups had a roentgenograph of medium or severe heart dilation, but there was only one case with obvious heart dilation in the treated group (Table 9-6). Physical examination and an electrocardiograph revealed more abnormalities of patients in the control than in the treated group, both in the beginning and in the ending examinations (Tables 9-7 and 9-8).

Similar work has been carried out in other provinces, covering

Table 9-5. Incidence Rate and Prognosis of Se Treated and Control Children in 1974–1977

Groups	Year	Subjects	Total Cases	Alive	Turned Latent	Cases Improved	Turned Chronic	Death
Control	1974	3985	54	27	16	9	2	27
	1975	5445	52	26	13	10	3	26
Treated	1974	4510	10	10	9	0	1	0
	1975	6767	7	6	6	0	0	1

Table 9-6. Heart X-Ray Examination of Se Treated and Control Children in 1974–1977

Groups	Year of Incidence	Cases	Year of Examination	Cases Examined	Normal[a]	Slight Dilation[a]	Moderate[a] Dilation	Severe Dilation[a]
Control	1974	54	1974	36	7[b]	—	29[b]	—
			1975	29	13	6	4	6
			1976	26	13	4	4	3
			1977	26	14	6	4	2
	1975	52	1975	35	11	4	10	10
			1976	25	12	4	5	4
			1977	25	9	10	5	1
Treated	1974	10	1974	8	2[b]	—	6[b]	—
			1975	9	7	1	0	1
			1976	9	7	1	0	1
			1977	10	8	1	0	1
	1975	7	1975	6	6	0	0	0
			1976	6	5	1	0	0
			1977	5	4	1	0	0

[a]Heart chest Ratio: normal 0.46–0.51; slight dilation 0.52–0.55; moderate dilation 0.56–0.60; severe dilation over 0.60.
[b]Examined by fluoroscopy; the results were divided into normal and dilated heart.

Table 9-7. Main Signs of Se Treated and Control Children in 1974–1977

Group	Year	Cases	Year of Examination	Cases Examined	Gallop Rhythm	Heart Failure	Cardiogenic Shock	Arrhythmia	Hemiplegia
Control	1974	54	1974	53	51	50	3	1	2
			1975	31	5	12	0	0	2
			1976	28	0	3	0	0	2
			1977	26	0	1	0	0	2
	1975	52	1975	52	48	47	4	3	0
			1976	28	0	7	0	0	0
			1977	25	2	1	0	1	0
Treated	1974	10	1974	10	10	9	0	0	0
			1975	10	1	1	0	0	0
			1976	10	0	1	0	0	0
			1977	10	0	1	0	0	0
	1975	7	1975	7	2	1	1	0	0
			1976	6	0	0	0	0	0
			1977	6	0	0	0	0	0

Table 9-8. The ECG changes of Se Treated and Control Children in 1974–1977

Groups	Year of Incidence	Cases	Year of Examination	Cases Examined	Normal	Low Volage	IRBBB	RBBB	IVB[a]	ST-T Change	A-V Block	VE[b]
Control	1974	54	1974	43	11	16	10	5	0	16	1	1
			1975	28	17	2	2	1	2	2	1	0
			1976	24	19	1	1	0	1	2	0	0
			1977	26	19	1	1	0	0	0	0	0
	1975	52	1975	38	5	12	6	9	0	18	3	2
			1976	24	15	3	3	3	0	4	0	0
			1977	24	16	1	2	3	0	0	0	0
Treated	1974	10	1974	10	6	2	3	0	0	0	0	0
			1975	10	7	1	3	0	1	0	0	0
			1976	9	6	0	2	0	1	0	0	0
			1977	10	6	0	3	0	1	0	0	0
	1975	7	1975	7	1	1	2	0	0	6	0	0
			1976	6	5	0	1	0	0	0	0	0
			1977	6	5	0	1	0	0	0	0	0

[a] Intraventricular block.
[b] Ventricular extrasystoles.

500,000 subjects. All the results confirmed the effectiveness of oral administration of sodium selenite against Keshan disease. No untoward side effects were reported. Physical examination and liver function tests were performed on 100 children who had taken selenium for 3 or 4 years. No significant difference was observed as compared with the control group children.

THE ETIOLOGY OF KESHAN DISEASE

Facts given above suggest strongly that selenium deficiency may play an important role in the occurrence of Keshan disease. However, there are still phenomena which cannot be explained by deficiency alone. The disease has a seasonal prevalence—winter in the north and summer in the south. Also, it presented peak incidence in certain years in some districts. However, the selenium content of grains and hair did not vary dramatically from year to year nor among seasons. Therefore, there should be another factor or factors involved in the etiology or pathogenesis of this disease. Viral infection seems to be the most notable one among the suspects.

A number of viral strains have been isolated from the blood, heart tissue, and other organs of the victims. Most of them are in the Echo or Coxsackie families (6). One strain, named CB-21, identified as Coxsackie virus B4, was obtained in 1974 from the blood sample of a 3½-year old boy who was suffering from subacute Keshan disease. The pathogenesis of this virus was tested with suckling mice in combination with selenium (7). Kunming 210 mice were divided into groups consuming different diets beginning 6 weeks before mating and continuing through the test. The control group consumed a stock feed containing 0.518 ppm of selenium; the test group, a feed containing 0.01 ppm of selenium mainly consisting of grains produced in the affected site. A third group took the same test feed with adequate selenium supplementation (as aqueous solution of sodium selenite, by esophageal intubation). The blood selenium levels of animals in different groups were well in agreement with their intake. They were 0.544 ppm in the control, 0.057 ppm in the test, and 0.302 ppm in the supplemented group.

Each baby mouse accepted 0.07 ml of virus culture intraperitoneally. All animals were injected in their seventh day of life and sacrificed 7 days after injection. The blood selenium levels of suckling mice are comparable to those of the adults. Pathological examination revealed myocardial

Table 9-9.   Blood Selenium Content and Heart Lesion of the Suckling Mice

Groups	Blood Se (ppm)	Animal Number	Myocardionecrosis		
			Cases	%	Average Severity[a]
Control	0.306	52	8	15	41
Supplemented	0.138	30	13	13	69
Test	0.010	56	20	36	119

[a] Number of microsquares occupied by the necrotic areas on the heart section, measured with a microgrid under microscope.

necrosis in association with their blood selenium contents. Both the frequency and the severity of heart damage of the test group roughly double those of the control group. The supplemented group, although they had the poor test diet, suffered as many heart lesions as the control group (Table 9-9). The difference between the deficient and adequate groups is statistically significant ($p < 0.01$). The pathological characteristics of the heart lesions of baby mice somewhat resemble those of Keshan disease.

In addition, electron microscopy revealed small unidentified particles in 7 of 11 observed Keshan disease cases. The particles are roughly round with a diameter of $20-27$ mμ and located in damaged myocardiocytes. The possibility of their being viral particles has not been ruled out.

All the results are tempting us to go further on exploring the possibility that the combination of selenium deficiency with viral infection might be the answer to the etiology of Keshan disease.

In summary:

1. Keshan disease is endemic in a wide belt in China.
2. The primary lesion is a multifocal necrosis of myocardium.
3. More than 10 million people are affected.
4. Selenium levels are low in people in affected areas.
5. The disease is prevented by prophylaxis with sodium selenite.
6. Animal studies suggest the possibility of a viral infection in a selenium-deficient subject.

Works in this presentation were carried out by all members of the Keshan Disease Research Team headed by Dr. Xiaoshu Chen, Dr. Keyou Ge, and Dr. Junshi Chen. Professor Guangqi Yang, Professor Xuecun Chen, Dr. Zhimei Wen, and Professor Lianzhen Zhu and group also took part in organizing and conducting these works. The Team consisted of persons from the Institute of Health, Fuwai Hospital, Institute of Pediatrics, and Capital Hospital of Chinese Academy of Medical Sciences.

These investigations were completed with the effective assistance of the health workers of the local health units in all areas involved, especially of the antiepidemic stations of Sichuan province, of Xichang prefecture, and Mianing county.

REFERENCES

1. K. Ge, A. Xue, and S. Wang, *Chinese Med. J.* (English Abstract), **60,** 407 (1980).
2. Keshan Disease Research Group of Chinese Academy of Medical Sciences, *Chinese Med. J.* (English Issue), **92,** 477 (1979).
3. J. B. Wilkie et al., *J. Agr. Food Chem.,* **18,** 945 (1970).
4. D. G. Hafman et al., *J. Nutr.,* **104,** 580 (1973).
5. Keshan Disease Research Group of Chinese Academy of Medical Sciences, *Chinese Med. J.* (English Issue), **92,** 471 (1979).
6. Chengqi Su et al., *Chinese Med. J.,* **59,** 466 (1979).
7. Bai Jin et al., *Acta Acad. Med. Sinicae* (English Abstract), **2,** 29 (1980).

10

Anorexia Nervosa

LESTER BAKER, M.D., AND KENNETH R. LYEN,
M.R.C.P.

School of Medicine, University of Pennsylvania

Anorexia nervosa probably represents one of the more frequent causes of malnutrition in adolescents living in developed countries. Although no firm data are available, it appears that both the absolute number and the frequency of patients with this syndrome have increased greatly over the past decade. The mortality rate at present in major treatment centers is of the order of 1 to 2% (1−3), rather than the 5 to 15% usually quoted in the older literature (4−9). In a disease that is potentially treatable, it is difficult to accept any mortality. Further improvement in the psychiatric treatment of anorexia nervosa is vital. Proper nutritional assessment and treatment of these patients would also be of major importance in reducing mortality.

However, when one turns to the published literature concerning the nutritional aspects of anorexia nervosa, one finds a striking paucity of relevant information. It is therefore necessary to start afresh, asking what the fundamental issues are, and how to approach these basic problems. From the nutritional point of view, the following questions are of prime importance in the patient with anorexia nervosa:

1. Several other forms of malnutrition have been studied extensively. Can lessons be drawn from these models which might be

Supported in part by RR 240 and MH 21336

applicable to the patient with anorexia nervosa? Are there nutritional deficiencies that are relatively specific for anorexia nervosa?

2. What causes death in patients with anorexia nervosa? How can one tell how close to death any given patient might be?
3. When starting nutritional rehabilitation:
    a. Which route should be used?
    b. Are there guidelines for the number of calories required and the distribution of those calories with regard to protein, carbohydrate, and fat?
4. How does one monitor the patient:
    a. In order to ensure the efficacy of therapy?
    b. To avoid any complications?

MODELS OF MALNUTRITION

It is tempting to take the studies of marasmus and kwashiorkor in children in developing countries as possible models for anorexia nervosa. One also turns to the classic studies of starvation in adult volunteers (the Minnesota experiments of Keys and co-workers), and to the observations made during famines in World War II (10,11) for further insights into what may be occurring in patients with anorexia nervosa. The first and perhaps the most formidable problem is that patients with anorexia nervosa comprise an extremely heterogeneous group. The clinical symptoms of these patients allow them to be grouped together under the syndrome of anorexia nervosa, using the criteria of Feighner and co-workers (12), but from the nutritional point of view they cover a vast array of potential abnormalities. Some patients may reduce calories drastically, but continue to eat a reasonable amount of protein. Others adopt very bizarre and idiosyncratic diets (one of our patients insisted that 2 slices of celery covered with ketchup constituted "a meal"). Some patients even restrict water intake. The abuse of laxatives or diuretics is also a clearly recognized pattern, as is that of eating followed by induced vomiting. It is extremely important to keep this heterogeneity in mind when one tries to make overly broad nutritional recommendations.

Although it is true that many patients with anorexia nervosa have a nutritional history that resembles the malnutrition seen in patients with marasmus and kwashiorkor, studies of these entities cannot be applied to patients with anorexia nervosa for three major reasons. Anorexia nervosa is generally regarded as a disease of early to middle adolescence.

Malnourished children from developing countries are usually much younger. Patients with anorexia nervosa usually start from a point of adequate nutrition before the onset of their psychiatric disease. The children with malnutrition from developing countries have often been undernourished throughout their lives. Children from developing countries who suffer from malnutrition often have other concomitant diseases (such as diarrhea and parasitic infestations), which complicate their nutritional state and their needs for nutritional rehabilitation.

The experiences during the famine in Leningrad (11) and Holland during World War II (10) are perhaps more nearly relevant. The major additional problems caused by wartime stresses and the destruction of sanitary and social services make these experiences not quite comparable. In addition, there are few complete studies, particularly concerning the documentation of specific deficiencies and the testing of different approaches to realimentation. This is understandable enough, given the chaotic social conditions present during a wartime phenomenon, but it still leaves us with little specific information.

The Minnesota experiments (10) conducted on healthy adult volunteers provide many interesting observations. Again, these do not contribute significantly to our understanding of anorexia nervosa because of the lack of comparability of the diets, as well as the key fact that the volunteers were not allowed to undergo the same order of weight loss as is often seen in patients with anorexia nervosa.

From the foregoing discussion, it is almost redundant to state that no deficiencies specific for anorexia nervosa have been identified. In part, this relates to the nutritional heterogeneity of the group. It also relates to the absence of studies in anorexia nervosa to document such important parameters as total body potassium, protein turnover rates, and abnormalities in the distribution of water between the intracellular and extracellular compartments. A recent abstract (13) which indicated that total body potassium was reduced to levels below 50% of expected in two patients is an example of the kind of information necessary before one can formulate a more rational approach to nutrition in these patients.

DEATH IN ANOREXIA NERVOSA

Table 10-1 presents a summary of the causes of death in patients with anorexia nervosa obtained from major papers over the past 15 years (1–9). Several important points emerge:

142

Table 10-1. Causes of Death in Anorexia Nervosa

First Author	Year of Publication	Total Number of Patients	Number Died	Percentage Died	Cause Not Known or "Starvation"	Suicide	Low Plasma Potassium	Hypoglycaemia	Infection	Cardiopulmonary	Iatrogenic	Other
Seidensticker	1968	60	9	15%	3	2		1	2			1 (brain tumor)
Browning	1968	36	3	8%							2	1 (asthma)
Dally	1969	140	4	3%	3	1						
Theander	1970	94	12	13%		3			"some"	"some"		1 (bleeding from tooth extract'n)
Bruch	1971	64	4	6%	2		1					1 (calcinosis, heart, renal)
Morgan	1975	41	2	5%		1						1 (asthma)
Garfinkel	1977	42	1	2%		1						
Hsu	1979	100	2	2%			1				1	2 (electrolyte disturbances)
Pertschuk	in press	77	1	1%								
Total (percentage)		654	38	5.8%	8(21%)	8(21%)	1(3%)	1(3%)	2+	+	3(8%)	7(18%)

1. The reports are grossly deficient. In some reports, absence of good clinical monitoring and the lack of postmortem studies render the data incomplete and potentially misleading. For example, how can one deal with the conclusion that unspecified "electrolyte disturbances" caused death in two patients in the series of Hsu et al. (2)? In some reports, an attempt to define a specific cause of death may also be misleading. Given the general clinical experience, it is hard to know how much weight to give to the conclusion that hypoglycemia or infection caused death.

2. A significant percentage (21%) of patients committed suicide.

3. Iatrogenetic causes are listed in this table as being responsible for 8% of the total deaths. This probably is an underestimate of the true number. It is extremely important to keep in mind that "iatrogenesis imperfecta" can be a lethal disease.

When one turns from a general analysis of the causes of death to the problems of a specific patient, one is always confronted with the issue of deciding how close to the "point of no return" any given patient may be. The answer to this question will obviously influence one of the major early clinical decisions: namely, how much time is available to push a specific psychiatric regimen, while accepting lack of improvement in the nutritional area. Although this area is poorly studied, there are several candidates that might serve as prognostic indicators of potential high mortality risk. The following list is offered, based on personal observations and an analysis of reports of death in the literature:

1. History of laxative or diuretic abuse, or bizarre dietary intake. This might cause the patient to be highly vulnerable to potential electrolyte problems.

2. Physical findings:
    a. Less than 50% of ideal body weight. In 13 patients in the series of causes of death in anorexia, sufficient information was available to assess the degree of weight loss at the time of death. The mean weight loss was 51.8%, with a standard error of 3.6%. The degree of weight loss seen in the survivors in those series was, unfortunately, not given; hence drawing a definitive conclusion is difficult. Dally(6) has noted much the same and has suggested that a weight loss greater than 50% of ideal weight is strongly associated with an increased risk for mortality.

    b.   Marked hypothermia (less than 95°F). Many patients with anorexia nervosa adapt to their state of malnutrition with a lowered body temperature. A more marked degree is suggestive of the possibility of rapid deterioration.

    c.   Hypotension. Although blood pressure in most patients with anorexia nervosa is lower, one should be particularly concerned about those individuals whose age-adjusted blood pressure shows marked lowering, or who demonstrate postural hypotension. The potential for cardiovascular collapse in any of these patients is a point to bear in mind. In addition to volume depletion, starvation is known to be associated with a cardiomyopathy of undetermined cause (14).

    d.   Mental status changes suggestive of a toxic encephalopathy. Patients with anorexia nervosa are well known to have bizarre body image distortions and often complusive behavior with regard to food. The presence of other changes may be associated with a degree of malnutrition that would be extremely dangerous to the patient.

3.   Laboratory evidence of:

    a.   Low serum potassium or electrocardiographic abnormalities. Hypokalemia is quite common in anorexia nervosa but has been implicated as the cause of death in only two reports. This no doubt represents an underestimate of the importance of this problem. Serum potassium level is a late index of potassium depletion. A reduction in total potassium of the order of 50%, as found in preliminary work by Crosby and co-workers (13), would clearly render the patient highly vulnerable to acute changes, particularly during the period of realimentation.

    b.   Hypoglycemia. Asymptomatic hypoglycemia is relatively common but has been ascribed as a cause of death in two papers. The presence of hypoglycemia in some ways might relate to a deficiency of gluconeogenetic substrate, and thus raises concerns about whether the patient's protein stores are close to complete exhaustion.

    c.   Absence of ketonuria despite starvation. In a patient who is taking no calories, the absence of ketonuria may be ominous. Normally, in prolonged fasting, ketone bodies derived from adipose tissue lipolysis and hepatic ketogenesis serve as an alternative fuel for the brain. Absence of ketone bodies might therefore reflect such severe inanition that virtually all adipose tissue stores have been depleted. There also appears to be a relationship between ketone body elevation and suppression of protein breakdown. A fall in ketone bodies might therefore signal an accelerated rate of protein breakdown, and be of disastrous consequences.

NUTRITIONAL REHABILITATION

The initial phases of therapy with the anorectic must focus on the life-threatening syndrome. The child must begin to eat and to regain weight. We have tended to use a combination of behavioral interventions and family therapy techniques specifically directed toward the presenting problem, which can usually achieve symptom remission in a few weeks (15). Before putting these measures into action, however, the pediatrician must decide whether the patient presents a nutritional emergency, using the guidelines suggested in the previous table. In such a case, vigorous supportive nutritive and caloric therapy will be necessary. Any attempts at psychiatric therapy (including the behavioral modification program) should be deferred until the patient is nutritionally reconstituted to the point where she is no longer in danger. Psychotherapy with a patient who is toxic is both dangerous and ineffective.

One of the initial decisions may be whether the patient should be considered a candidate for intravenous hyperalimentation, an approach currently receiving attention (16), or whether nasogastric tube feedings should be commenced. A rational nutritional choice between these two should be made on the basis of knowledge of gastrointestinal function in patients with anorexia nervosa.

Although the number of studies has been small, it appears that gastrointestinal structure and function are intact in patients with anorexia nervosa. Gastric peristolic activity appears to be normal, as is small intestinal peristalsis, in patients with anorexia nervosa who are not taking laxatives (17, 18). Barium studies of the gastrointestinal tract in eight patients were found to be normal (19). In a small number of patients in whom intestinal biopsy was performed, no structural changes in the small intestine were found (19). While Silverman et al. found an abnormality of xylose absorption (20), other studies have been performed in which both lactose tolerance and fat absorption have been found to be normal in patients with anorexia nervosa (19, 21). There thus appears to be no defined abnormality in the gastrointestinal system of the patient with anorexia nervosa which would preclude alimentation by mouth.

There appears to be considerable heterogeneity in the anorectic group in terms of the food which they will consume. Both Dally (6) and Russell (22) noted that most of their patients were quite selective in their choice of foods, generally tending to avoid starchy foods and thus reduce carbohydrate content. Both also noted a relatively increased protein intake. On the other hand, in the study by Marshall (23), carbohydrate intake was not preferentially restricted; these patients drastically reduced their total caloric intake.

The caloric requirements for patients with anorexia nervosa may be underestimated if one uses only resting energy expenditure, as derived by indirect calorimetry (13). Russell and Mezey (24) suggested a mean caloric intake of 75 cal/kg for weight gain during treatment for anorexia nervosa; this was confirmed by Walker and colleagues (25). Marshall (23) allowed a group of 17 patients with anorexia nervosa free access to a variety of food. Four of these patients ate 70% or more of their recommended caloric intake and gained weight. Of the remaining 13 who ate less than that, 11 continued to lose weight, while 2 managed to sustain their already low body weights.

Just as there exists a shortage of studies on the absolute nutritional requirements in these patients, there are almost no observations concerning the optimal composition of the nutritional program. In studies of protein turnover in malnourished children (26), protein catabolism was reduced to a greater extent if, upon refeeding, the intake consisted of a high carbohydrate content when compared to one with a high protein content. It is known from human volunteer studies that carbohydrate can reduce gluconeogenesis and therefore has a protein sparing effect (27). In the only study in anorexia nervosa, one patient showed no significant differences in protein synthesis at two different levels of protein and caloric intake (28). This result seems most unusual and warrants repeating.

In summary, there are no known contraindications to the use of the patient's own gastrointestinal tract for nutritional rehabilitation. Initial attempts at oral feeding should emphasize easily absorbed carbohydrate but not to the exclusion of protein. Calculations can be made using 60 to 75 cal/kg as a reasonable starting point.

MONITORING

It is important to state the obvious: patients must be monitored closely not only to ensure the efficacy of a given regimen, but also to avoid potential problems. Clearly it is important to follow those parameters associated with an increased mortality risk. Thus, improvements in body temperature, blood pressure, and pulse should be documented. Similarly, any abnormalities of potassium, phosphorus, and glucose should be corrected. Problems concerning potassium and phosphate may be unmasked during the early phases of realimentation, and these must be watched most carefully. In the initial stages of nutritional rehabilitation, it is not clear whether weight gain reflects mostly fluid retention or actual gain in body mass. Nonetheless, it is clear that weight should proceed in the proper direction.

CLINICAL IMPLICATIONS

In medicine, one attempts to achieve a specific diagnosis and then to formulate a rational approach to therapy. In the patient with anorexia nervosa, this may not be simple and straightforward. Nonetheless, the observations that have been reviewed in this presentation do have several major clinical implications. These may be summarized as follows:

1. Patients with anorexia nervosa are an extremely heterogeneous group. The state of preceding nutrition, the nature of the idiosyncratic diet adopted by a specific patient, the possible restriction of water intake, and the possible abuse of laxatives and diuretics can all play an important role in the nutritional state of the patient as she presents for evaluation and treatment.

2. Patients who are at the highest risk for possible death can be identified through a constellation of historical traits, physical findings, and laboratory examinations. These patients require immediate intervention to correct any tendency to cardiovascular collapse or to electrolyte abnormalities. However, after that point, the nutritional approach to these patients has to be "conservatively aggressive." Although changes need to be made, these patients have often achieved a very delicate balance which can be easily altered for the worse. Thus, the intervention must be graduated, and the patient must be monitored extremely carefully. The more vigorous and the more unphysiologic the intervention, the closer the patient needs to be monitored, and the more likely it is that the patient will fall victim to "iatrogenesis imperfecta."

3. All patients should be closely evaluated as to their suicidal potential.

4. The patient's own gastrointestinal tract is the most physiological route for nutritional rehabilitation. The current interest in intravenous hyperalimentation should be viewed with great caution.

5. It is important to have a team approach to these patients. They have a psychiatric disease that is life threatening because of its nutritional aspects. The psychiatrist and the pediatrician/internist must have their specific roles defined. The nutritional evaluation and all nutritional decisions should be made by the pediatrician/internist. When the psychiatrist pushes for a delay in nutritional rehabilitation in order to give more time for the program to work, or when the pediatrician/internist becomes embroiled in the workings of the behavioral modification paradigm, it is the patient who gets placed in a vulnerable position. The decision around hyperalimentation may sometimes blur the therapeutic roles of pediatrician/internist and psychiatrist. If the psychiatrist prefers the intravenous route because of the assessment of the patient's fear of rape or pregnancy, that should be stated clearly, and not masked in terms of nutritional needs.

6. There is a great need in this field for sophisticated studies with regard to such important issues as total body potassium, total body water and its compartmentation, and methods of evaluation of protein and lipid stores. These studies would help in the classification of nutritional risk in different patients within this heterogeneous group of anorexia nervosa. It could thus lead to the desired aim of a more specific and rational therapeutic program for each individual patient.

REFERENCES

1. P. E. Garfinkel, H. Moldofsky, and D. N. Gardner, *Canad. Med. Assn. J.*, **117**, 1041 (1977).

2. L. K. G. Hsu, A. H. Crisp, and B. Harding, *Lancet*, **I**, 61 (1979).

3. M. J. Pertschuk, J. Forster, G. Buzby, and J. L. Mullen, The treatment of anorexia nervosa with total parenteral nutrition. (In press).

4. J. F. Seidensticker and M. Tzagournis, *J. Chron. Dis.*, **21**, 361 (1968).

5. C. H. Browining and S. I. Miller, *Am. J. Psychiat.*, **124**, 1128 (1968).

6. P. Dally, *Anorexia Nervosa*, Heinemann, London, 1969.

7. S. Theander, *Acta Psychiat. Scand.* (Suppl.), **214**, 1 **(1970)**.

8. H. Bruch, *Psychosomatic Med.*, **33**, 135 (1971).

9. H. C. Morgan and G. F. M. Russell, *Psychol. Med.*, **5**, 355 (1975).

10. A. Keys, J. Brozek, A. Henschel, *The Biology of Human Starvation*, University of Minnesota Press, 1950.

11. J. Brozek, A. Wells, and A. Keys, *Am. Rev. Sov. Med.*, **4**, 70 (1946).

12. J. P. Feighner, E. Robins, S. B. Guze, et al., *Arch. Gen. Psych.*, **26**, 57 (1972).

13. I. Feurer, L. Crosby, M. J. Pertschuk, and J.Mullen, *J. Parenteral Enteral Nutr.* (1980).

14. J. S. Gottdiener, H. A. Gross, W. L. Henry, J. S. Bover, and M. H. Ebert, *Circulation*, **58**, 425 (1978).

15. S. Minuchin, B. Rosman, and L. Baker, *Psychosomatic Families: Anorexia Nervosa in Context*, Harvard University Press, Cambridge, 1978.

16. B. A. Finkelstein, *J.A.M.A.*, **219**, 217 (1972).

17. A. H. Crisp, *Proc. R. Soc. Med.*, **58**, 814 (1965).

18. J. T. Silverstone and G. F. M. Russell, *Br. J. Psychiat.*, **113**, 257 (1967).

19. J. D. Gryboski, J. Katz, M.H. Sangree, and T. Herskovic, *Clin. Pediatr.*, **7**, 684 (1968).

20. J. A. Silverman, "Anorexia Nervosa: Clinical and Metabolic Observations in a Successful Treatment Plan," in R. A. Vigersky, Ed., *Anorexia Nervosa*, Raven Press, New York, 1977, p. 331.

21. A. H. Crisp, *World Rev. Nutr. Dietetics*, **12**, 452 (1970).

22. G. F. M. Russell, M. Shepherd, and D. L. Davies, *Studies in Psychiatry*, Oxford Medical Publications, 1968.

23. M. H. Marshall, *J. Human Nutr.*, **32**, 349 (1978).

24. G. F. M. Russell, and A. G. Mezey, *Med. Sci.*, **23**, 449 (1962).

25. J. Walker, S. L. Roberts, K. A. Halmi, and S. C. Goldberg, *Am. J. Clin. Nutr.*, **32**, 1396 (1979).

26. M. Golden, J. C. Waterlow, and D. Picou, *Am. J. Clin. Nutr.*, **30**, 1345 (1977).

27. O. E. Owen, P. Felig, A. P. Morgan, J. Wahren, G. F. Cahill, Jr., *J. Clin. Invest.*, **48**, 574 (1969).

28. A. Kassenaar, J. deGraeff, and A. T. Kouwenhoven, *Metabolism*, **9**, 831 (1960).

11

Adolescent Obesity

JEROME L. KNITTLE, M.D., KIM I. TIMMERS, Ph. D.,
AND DAVID P. KATZ, Ph.D.

Mount Sinai School of Medicine, New York, New York

Obesity is a common nutritional problem and is associated with increased risk, and complication, of a number of life-threatening conditions. In addition, mortality figures indicate that obese patients have a shorter life expectancy and are subject to more surgical and obstetrical complications, including those causing death, than their nonobese counterparts. Although transitory amelioration of the obese state can be achieved, the long-term treatment of this disorder has been uniformly disappointing, and after weight reduction obese adults rapidly regain their former weight once caloric restriction ends (1−9).

The failure of obese adults to maintain the reduced state may be because dietary intervention usually occurs after the morphological and metabolic factors that contribute to the obese state are well established. If reduced weights are to be maintained, the obese adult must resign himself or herself to the fact that caloric restriction must be continued after the desired weight loss has been achieved.

Indeed the treatment of obesity in humans has been largely limited to one form or another of caloric restriction after the development of the disorder. In general, the success of these programs is measured by the amount of weight lost and the ease, or the speed, with which ideal weight is achieved. Little, if any, attention is paid to the long-term consequences, which are almost universally disappointing. Furthermore, one of the major shortcomings in the treatment of obese subjects is our lack of a clear-cut definition of obesity. The point at which the body fat of an individual and particularly of a child or adolescent becomes sufficiently excessive to warrant a diagnosis of obesity is difficult to define. Many mathematical models and indices have been developed to identify obese individuals. Some have used 20–25% above ideal weight in children. In the adult, one can use terminology of percent fat, so that if 40% or more of one's body weight is fat one would be defined as an obese adult. Data for children and adolescents are less precise. In adolescents it would depend upon what age and what stage of adolescence the child is in; is the child developing or has the child reached full growth?

One other measure used is to assess subcutaneous fat by means of skinfold thickness. This measurement provides an additional means to account for variations in weight due to increased muscle mass or heavy bony skeleton. For adolescent boys the normal mean skinfold is 18 mm at age 12 decreasing to 14 mm at age 17, then gradually increasing in the late teens to 18 mm at age 22. Girls show a constant rise from 23 mm at 14 years, to 26 mm at 17, to 28 mm at 22.

A more reasonable approach would be to develop methods for easily determining total body fat in the adolescent. Our approach has been to look at the obese individual from the point of view of cellular development of the adipose tissue and its relation to total body weight. The issues we have considered are why certain individuals develop abnormal growth patterns of adipose tissue which result in obesity. Are there determining factors in the development of obesity? Are they genetic or environmental? Do metabolic and/or endocrine dysfunction cause, or are they a sequel to, obesity?

To answer these questions we have attempted to develop techniques that might be useful in identifying the obesity-prone individual so that a rational approach to the prevention of obesity might be developed. Studies of adipose depot development in humans have been stimulated by the methodology of Hirsch and Gallian (10). The method is limited first by the fact that only cells with some lipid content can be identified. Those cells that are either depleted of their fat stores or destined to store lipid at some future date cannot be counted, since the sole identifying characteristic of the adipocyte is the presence of fat. However, given these shortcomings, the technique has been useful in defining the cellular characteristics of obese and nonobese subjects and in clarifying data relating metabolic function to cellularity.

In our laboratory we have been interested in cellular development of the fat depot and have instituted longitudinal studies of the fat depot in children ranging from 4 months to 16 years of age. The technique of needle aspiration was used (10). The procedure is simple and safe, even in children. One anesthetizes the subcutaneous area with 1–2 ml of 1%

xylocaine, then inserts a 15-gauge needle attached to a siliconized 50-ml glass syringe. When one pulls back on the plunger, the fat tissue issues forth by suction. As much as 500 mg of fat can be removed with each sampling. Fat cell number was determined by dividing the average fat cell size into a value for total body fat, which was derived from the measurement of total body K^+. This technique is limited by the fact that we were unable to measure total body K^+ in children under 2 years of age because of the lack of sensitivity of the counter. Thus, results in children younger than 2 are based on height–weight relationships. Two groups of subjects were studied: obese subjects over 130% of ideal body weight and nonobese subjects between 90% and 120% of ideal weight. From 2 to 16 years of age no significant differences in cell size were observed between children of different ages in obese subjects. In nonobese subjects, cell size also showed no difference with age from 2 to 10; however, after this time cell size was significantly larger in obese children when compared to fat cells from nonobese children of the same age. However, the differences in size were not statistically significant after 12 years of age. Furthermore, at 2 years of age, obese children displayed cell sizes within the adult range of 0.4–0.7 μg lipid/cell, whereas nonobese subjects did not achieve adult levels until after age 12 (Figure 11-1).

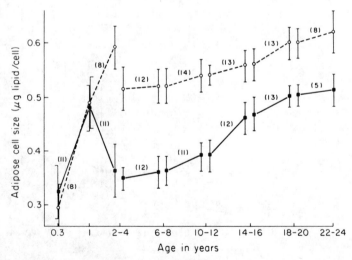

Figure 11-1.   Longitudinal studies of adipose cell size as a function of age in years. Obese subjects are represented as open circles and nonobese as black squares. (n) = number of subjects studied at each 4-year interval. Each point represents mean values ± SEM.

Differences in adipose cell number were also found. Significant differences in cell number were detected as early as 2 years of age and persisted throughout the entire range studied. Obese subjects displayed increases in cell number in all ages. However, no change in cell number was observed in nonobese subjects between 2 and 12 years of age. Once again increments in this factor were found only after age 12 (Figure 11-2).

Thus, after 2 years of age one can detect significant quantitative as well as qualitative differences in adipose tissue growth and development between obese and nonobese children. Obese children attained adult levels for fat cell size by age 2 and thereafter increased their fat stores almost exclusively by increases in cell number. Nonobese subjects displayed a relative quiescence in adipose depot enlargement from 2 years of age until prepubescent and adolescent periods. At that time both cell size and number appeared to increase.

We have also followed children from 4 months to 4 years of age. Fat aspirations were repeated at 6- to 8-month intervals prior to age 12 and at yearly intervals thereafter. Eight of the subjects studied clinically developed overt obesity. The data obtained from these individuals during the course of our observation were matched with subjects of comparable age and sex who did not become obese. No significant differences in weight were observed prior to and up to 12 months of age.

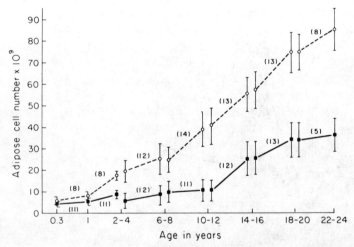

Figure 11-2. Longitudinal studies of adipose cell number as a function of age in years. Obese subjects are represented as open circles and nonobese as black squares. (*n*) = number of subjects at 4-year interval. Each point represents mean values ± SEM.

Indeed, although not statistically significant, the mean weight of the subsequently obese children was less than that observed in the nonobese at birth and 4 months of age. However by 24 months of age, the obese group was significantly heavier, with a mean weight of 18.8 kg compared to 13.0 kg in the nonobese, and they remained heavier until 4 years of age. In both groups cell number continued to increase throughout the study. Although obese subjects display a greater number of cells at all ages, the differences were not statistically significant until 24 months of age (Figure 11-2). Thus, one could not clearly distinguish between obese and nonobese children on the basis of either total cell number or rate of cellular development at any time under 24 months of age. From 4 to 12 months of age both groups showed significant increments in lipid content and one could not distinguish the groups on the basis of size at either of these ages (Figure 11-1). However, from 12 to 24 months of age, whereas obese children continued to display significant increases in lipid content, nonobese subjects displayed a decrease, and by 24 months had a mean cell size that was significantly less than the obese child and smaller than that observed at 12 months of age.

Thus, although concrete evidence for "critical periods" or "set points" in adipose tissue development has not been demonstrated, the cellular data compiled to date suggest that two intervals in the development of adipose tissue may have important consequences for the development of obesity in man. The first period extends from birth to 2 years of age, and the second occurs somewhere in the prepubescent–pubescent period, stretching from about age 10–12 to 16. In both periods alterations in both cell number and size occur in nonobese subjects, some of whom may later become obese. Since alterations in cell size are intimately related to nutritional and hormonal factors, one could, perhaps, develop techniques to identify enzymatic markers or histochemical techniques that identify important precursor cells.

The early adipocyte enlargement found in obese children could be due to inherent differences in the fat cell of obese children, which results in abnormal response to normal hormonal influences, or to an altered hormonal milieu, which causes an increase in fat deposition or a decrease in lipolytic activity in the fat cell of the obese child.

These anatomical findings are consistent with *in vitro* metabolic studies of the response of adipose tissue from obese and nonobese subjects to the lipolytic effect of epinephrine. We have shown a diminished response to the lipolytic effect of this hormone in cells derived from obese subjects regardless of age (Figure 11-3). After weight reduction this diminished response does not change.

Since epinephrine is a major hormone in producing lipolysis in the fat

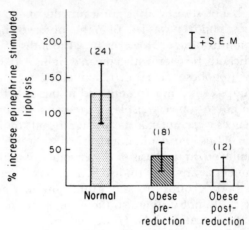

Figure 11-3. Percent increase over basal activity due to epinephrine stimulation in nonobese and obese subjects. *(n)* = number of subjects studied. Each point represent mean values ± SEM.

cell it is tempting to postulate an etiological role in the development of the hypercellularity and increased cell size found in obese subjects. The fact that its action appears not to be influenced by weight loss is further support for a primary role in the pathogenesis of this condition. Indeed, if a genetic obesity does exist in man, it could manifest itself in the form of altered enzymatic activity. One could speculate that the lack of epinephrine response serves as a stimulus for the development of new adipose cells. Thus a decrease in fatty acid released secondary to epinephrine stimulation in less responsive cells could result in an increased number of cells to meet energy needs. Since epinephrine action is mediated through the adenyl cyclase/cAMP system, one could postulate a defect there or in the protein kinase system.

Another area of research currently in progress in our laboratory is the study of specific enzymes of adipose tissue related to lipogenesis and glycolysis. We have measured levels of phosphofructokinase (PFK), malic enzyme (ME), and citrate cleavage enzyme (CCE) in adipose tissue from obese and nonobese subjects during weight maintenance, weight loss, and during refeeding.

The pattern of change with diet in several enzyme activities was different in obese versus nonobese subjects. The format used emphasizes the similarity within groups in the pattern of change with diet, rather than the difference in absolute values among individuals. As is shown on the right of Figure 11-4, CCE in nonobese subjects tended to decrease after a week of semistarvation. After 4 days of refeeding, CCE

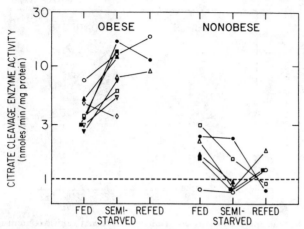

Figure 11-4.   Citrate cleavage enzyme activity as a function of dietary caloric content in obese and nonobese human adipose tissue. Abscissa is an arbitrary scale which serves to separate data obtained on different diets. Different symbols represent different individual subjects, each of whom was studied on more than one diet. Obese and nonobese subjects represented by the same symbol are not the same subject. The dashed line represents the limit of detection of the assay; symbols plotted below this line represent undetectable activity.

activity rebounded toward or beyond the previous "fed" levels in three out of five nonobese subjects but continued to fall in two others. In obese subjects, in contrast, CCE activity actually increased in seven out of eight subjects during weight loss ("semistarved") as compared to weight-maintenance ("fed"), $p < .05$. In three obese subjects studied after 4 days of refeeding, mean CCE activity was similar to that reached during semistarvation.

Malic enzyme activity (shown in Figure 11-5) was decreased during semistarvation in most obese and nonobese subjects and showed a refeeding rebound in some subjects. However, these trends were not statistically significant in either obese or nonobese groups. Phosphofructokinase activity (Figure 11-6) in nonobese subjects did not change significantly during semistarvation and refeeding. In seven out of eight obese subjects, in contrast, PFK activity increased about twofold during semistarvation as compared to the fed state ($p < .05$ for difference by diet, eight subjects). Phosphofructokinase activity tended to remain high after 4 days of refeeding in obese subjects.

These results were not dependent on the mode of presentation of the data; similar results were obtained when the data were expressed as activity per 10^6 fat cells.

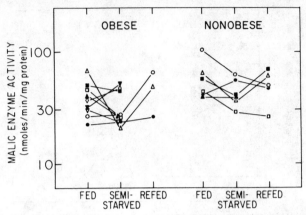

Figure 11-5. Malic enzyme activity as a function of dietary caloric content in obese and nonobese human adipose tissue. Abscissa and symbols as described in Figure 11-4.

The results show that in human adipose tissue, the activities of certain enzymes of glucose metabolism vary with the antecedent diet of the subject, and that the pattern of change with diet differs in obese versus nonobese individuals. In obese subjects, PFK and CCE activities tended to increase during semistarvation. In nonobese humans, in contrast, there were no effects of semistarvation and subsequent refeeding on PFK and CCE activity. These differences between obese and nonobese subjects in the response to semistarvation and refeeding suggest that different diet-induced signals, or different tissue response to similar endocrine or metabolic signals, may exist in the obese versus the nonobese individual.

The effects of low-calorie diets were discernible after 4 to 7 days in lean subjects and after 7 or more days in obese subjects. The pattern of change in activities in obese subjects did not appear to depend on the length of the period of semistarvation or on the degree of overweight, age at onset of obesity, or chronological age of the subject in the range of 9 to 45 years. Other work indicates that CCE and PFK activities are somewhat higher at 3 days and continue to increase in obese human adipose tissue at 7, 14, and 21 days of semistarvation as compared to the fed state; the activities remain elevated after several months of semistarvation.

We suggest that the increased CCE and PFK activities may reflect a metabolic adaptation to the semistarved state in obese subjects which is different from the adaptation produced in nonobese adipose tissue. This putative abnormality in the pattern of enzyme regulation in obesity

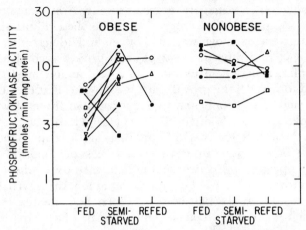

Figure 11-6. Phosphofructokinase activity as a function of dietary caloric content in obese and nonobese human adipose tissue. Abscissa and symbols as described in Figure 11-4.

might contribute to the rapid regain of weight that frequently occurs at the end of weight reduction programs and could provide an early marker for identification of the obesity-prone subject.

At present it appears that the growth of fat depots in humans is a result of complex interaction involving morphologic, genetic, metabolic, and nutritional factors. The degree to which any individual is susceptible to the effect of any one of these factors has not been determined to date. Whether or not all children may be prone to hypercellular states by overeating or whether overeating is a result of a genetic predisposition is currently unknown. However, our data suggest that some individuals can develop hypercellularity very early in life whereas others do so at a later date but prior to adolescence. Thus, one must be alert to the rapidly growing child whose weight outstrips his linear growth. Indeed, our findings suggest that once fat cell number is established, it cannot be decreased. However, nutritional factors instituted at the proper time may modify the rate of fat cell development in humans.

At present we do not have the definitive means to identify the obesity-prone child and are not even in agreement about the extent of the problem in children and adolescents or about the long-term consequences of being an obese child. Our cellular metabolic data indicate that for the grossly obese it is an unhappy future. Thus one is well advised to attack the problem early.

Figures representing the problem of obesity in adolescents range from 12.5% in teenage girls and 9.5% in teenage boys up to about 30%

of the population of teenagers in urban society. Approximately 80% of obese adolescents and children grow up to be obese adults and 25% of obese adults were once overweight children and adolescents.

Adolescence is a time of rapid physical growth second only to the prenatal infancy period in its rate. Since caloric and most nutritional needs tend to parallel the growth rate, it is obvious that the adolescents' needs are higher in proportion to body size than those of younger or older people. In 1932, Wait and Roberts (11) in a careful study of total energy needs of girls age 10–16 found that caloric requirements rose to a peak just before puberty at an average age of about 13 and then dropped. Eppright and co-workers (12) in a study of diets of school children in Iowa in the early 1950's also found that the girls had reached their peak caloric intake at about 12 years; boys on the other hand reached their maximum intake at about 11 years of age. In 1913, Heald et al. (13) confirmed the observation that maximum growth is likely to occur just before puberty and then to decline rapidly. Obviously before embarking on a dietary regimen one should assess the nutritional state of the patient and such things as hemoglobin and thyroid function, and, where indicated, vitamin levels should be obtained. In a study in California (14) of 127 teenagers, 15% of the girls failed to meet two-thirds of the recommended daily allowances for vitamins A and C while 10% of the boys failed to meet this level for vitamin A and 30% for vitamin C. Half the girls were low in iron and calcium, that is, less than two-thirds of recommended daily allowances. Even though 10% of the boys and girls consumed less than two-thirds the allowance of calories, obesity was not uncommon. Wharton (15) studying teenagers in three high schools in Southern Illinois, on the basis of 3-day diet records, reported a generally lower nutrient intake than in the Berkeley study and a far higher proportion of boys and girls who failed to meet two-thirds of the recommended allowances. However, we really have no information on the nutritional status of American teenagers as a whole and studies of the various groups indicate a tremendous variation in the level of nutritional status as well as degrees of obesity and caloric intake and incidence of obesity. Indeed we also lack good long-term data related to the number of obese adolescents that remain obese in adult life.

The most conservative estimates are that 50–65% of obese children remain obese through adulthood. The extent to which a group of these obese adults becomes at-risk for vascular and metabolic diseases is not readily apparent. Indeed one lacks a clear definition of obesity and its pathological implications. In her follow-up studies of children with obesity, Hilda Bruch has reported the outcome related to weight, personality adjustment, and results of various kinds of treatment (16, 17). Bruch followed an unselected group of 200 fat children, some for over 30 years, who were first evaluated for a variety of complaints, few of which were just obesity. The majority of patients were more than 50% overweight. Both overeating and inactivity were reported in 80%, with a high correlation between activity and emotional disturbances. Fewer than two-thirds of the group outgrew the condition during adolescence and were both well adjusted and slim. More than half of Bruch's group remained obese. A large number of these had serious adjustment problems and emotional illness. Thus even without any primary medical implications the psychosocial consequences of adolescent obesity in our society are profound and depressing and deserve to be treated.

The initial steps in the management of the obese child, adolescent, or adult are, as previously noted, a medical history and careful physical examination. Family histories of diabetes, hypertension, obesity, and vascular disease should be noted. A baseline diet history of the child and an inventory of the family dietary patterns are necessary for later alterations of caloric intake. Traditionally an assessment of parental interest and potential supportive measures within the family is useful. The medical history and physical examination with attention to blood pressure, duration and degree of obesity, and state of pubertal development generally differentiates exogenous obesity from the relatively uncommon disorders of thyroid dysfunction and adrenal dysfunction. There are a few uncommon childhood syndromes associated with obesity, such as: (1) Laurence Moon Biedl syndrome, with obesity, mental retardation, hypogonadism, polydactyly, retinitis pigmentosa, and renal disease; (2) Prader-Willis syndrome, consisting of obesity, hypogonadism, mental retardation, and hypotonia; and (3) Carpenter syndrome, with mental retardation, hypogonadism, polydactyly, and acrocephaly. The association in these syndromes of obesity with gonadal dysfunction and mental retardation suggests a hypothalamic defect. In the absence of any clinical suspicion of an underlying endocrine or genetic defect, further laboratory evaluation should be done to the extent appropriate to each individual. In subjects with a family history of diabetes and/or severe obesity one should get a glucose tolerance test with blood sugar and insulin determinations. Children who are hypertensive should receive hypertensive evaluation investigating for any primary cause of their hypertension. Thyroid function tests have not been helpful in our experience; however, they should be done at least to convince the parents and/or child that they are not dealing with a "glandular" disorder. Once known medical causes have been ruled out, we have our patient keep a dietary history using behavior modification techniques sheets. Although behavior modification approaches may not be useful in all individuals, we have found this form of data collection to be very useful in evaluating and delineating food intake, patterns of food intake, degree of hunger, emotional problems, and area within house and/or public domain that have high levels of food intake. Once these have been established, the caloric recommendations are made.

In discussing the treatment of obesity it is necessary to re-emphasize that one is dealing with a syndrome rather than a disease. The physician must be acquainted with the metabolic and psychological complexities of human obesity in order to deal better with this perplexing and frustrating problem. The concept of the obese subject as one who merely overindulges because of a lack of self-discipline can no longer be accepted.

The treatment of obesity is at once the simplest and yet the most complex of all disorders—simple in that, in the adult, all that is required is caloric restriction, and complex in that cellular, metabolic, socioeconomic, cultural, and psychological factors all militate against the maintenance of the reduced state. Unfortunately, in our society only the weight reduction period is emphasized and the obese subject is exposed to an endless variety of weight-reduction programs, which include diets, drugs, hormones, hypnosis, psychotherapy, and surgical intervention.

Although drastic crash programs may be necessary in life-threatening situations, such as the Pickwickian syndrome, diabetes, hypertension, or coronary artery disease, they are usually not necessary in uncomplicated cases. Furthermore, they do not prepare either the patient or the physician for a life of continuous dietary control. The preoccupation of both the lay and the medical community with weight loss alone has fostered the neglect of the postreduction period, which is in fact the more difficult problem. Thus most obese subjects live in a vicious cycle of weight loss followed by weight gain, ad infinitum, going from one "cure" to another in search of a magic formula.

The fact is that success with any weight reduction program will always be short-lived if it is not followed with supportive therapy that includes nutritional information suited to the tastes and life-styles of the individual. One must make the subject aware of the fact that once his or her desired weight is achieved, some degree of caloric restriction must be maintained if the reaccumulation of fat is to be avoided.

Obesity is a complex disorder and merely lecturing the patient or instilling guilt feelings by the use of such phrases as "weak-willed" or "cheating" will only be counterproductive. Rather one must be sympathetic and understanding of the enormity of the problem confronting the obese subject after weight loss is achieved. No one dietary program can be used for all patients, and it is up to the physician to work closely with the patient to find a program that is suitable. Any caloric restriction program that provides sufficient protein and minerals without promoting excessive ketosis or undue hunger will suffice.

Preparations for the weight loss and maintenance period should be made well in advance. The patient must be made to understand that a decrease in weight is not a cure-all. Most of the psychological and social problems that the patient has attributed to obesity will remain, and indeed some degree of depression and anxiety will occur as the subject realizes this fact. At this time the physician must be prepared to emphasize the positive aspects of the weight loss, such as changes in body image and other medical and social benefits.

The use of drugs, such as amphetamines, is of little value in the long-range treatment of obesity and should be assiduously avoided. This is especially true in children and adolescents who are already exposed to a drug-oriented society. The introduction of yet another medically approved drug creates the risk of subsequent harm from misuse. The short-term gain provided by these drugs is far outweighed by the long-term losses. Indeed, the reliance upon initial easy weight loss therapies may interfere with the initiation of effective weight maintenance programs by misleading the patient in regard to the nature and extent of effective long-term treatment.

The problem of dietary control is even more complicated in children and growing adolescents. In the adult most organ systems have reached their ultimate size and cellular division is complete. Weight reduction can be achieved almost exclusively by a decrease in body fat with little or no decrease in lean body mass. However, in the child one must provide sufficient calories and protein to allow for the growth and development of lean body mass, while achieving a decrease in the fat depot. The extent to which any dietary regimen will be responsible for these changes will depend upon the age at which it is instituted and the individual's level of cellular development. Unfortunately, at present our knowledge of the interrelationship of cellular growth and development of the various organ systems in the body is incomplete. No one diet can be devised that will deny calories and protein to the fat depot while providing the necessary nutrients to other tissues. Thus one must be extremely cautious and ever alert in restricting calories in the earliest age groups, and normal linear growth rates must be monitored.

We have used the Recommended Dietary Allowance (RDA) as our guide for the intake of calories and minerals based on the child's ideal weight for height and age. Calories are distributed as 20% protein, 45% carbohydrate, and 35% fat. It should be noted, however, when using the

RDAs that they are levels of intake of essential nutrients considered in the judgment of the Food and Nutrition Board, on the basis of available scientific knowledge, to be adequate to meet the known nutritional needs of almost every, healthy person. In each age group, however, a number of factors need to be considered which are interrelated. The requirements depend upon: (1) variability of nutritional components; (2) absorption in mixed meal patterns; (3) utilization of the materials at the levels of the cell which are dependent upon hormonal activity and enzymatic activity; (4) the age and sex of the individual; (5) the activity that is needed for maintaining growth and energy needs; (6) body composition, (7) socioeconomic levels; (8) cultural and religious factors; (9) disease processes involved at that particular time; and finally (10) possible medications being used.

As in the adult, one must be aware of the psychological and social problems, especially with younger children who are most dependent upon their parents. Indeed, one cannot alter dietary patterns of obese children without an understanding of their social milieu and the full cooperation of the family and school.

Once dietary restriction is instituted, weight loss and linear growth must be carefully monitored. Calories can then be readily increased or decreased in terms of body composition rather than total body weight. Indeed, the maintenance of a constant weight with an increasing ratio of lean body mass to body fat with normal linear growth is a desirable result. Ideally, of course, one would like to provide a diet at a critical period in the cellular development of the fat depot, so that adipose cell number would be held constant or decreased with minimal effect on the cellularity of nonfat organs. Unfortunately, at the present time this cannot be done because we lack sufficient information. However, it is hoped that studies of adipose tissue cellularity and metabolism described above, coupled with frequent longitudinal examinations of the same subject, will provide the necessary data to accomplish this end.

The development of techniques for the earliest identification of abnormal development of the fat depot and the institution of therapeutic measures to alter the development of this tissue before immutable hypercellularity occurs offer the best hope for the treatment of obesity in both children and adults. What is needed is research in the area of detection. One must identify obesity-prone subjects prior to the development of hypercellular states so that dietary restriction is not indiscriminately practiced on all infants and adolescents. At present we lack a specific marker for the obesity-prone child and must rely on our clinical acumen and follow the growth and development of our patients in order to detect the earliest clues to any aberrant patterns.

REFERENCES

1. T. Bjerkedal, *Acta Med. Scand.*, **13,** 159 (1957).
2. P. C. Davidson, and M. J. Albrink, *Metabolism*, **14,** 1059 (1965).
3. S. K. Fineberg, *J. Am. Geriat. Soc.*, **14,** 463 (1966).
4. A. Kagan, W. B. Kannel, T. R. Dawber, and N. Revotskie, *Ann. N. Y. Acad. Sci.*, **97,** 883 (1963).
5. L. H. Newburgh, and J. W. Conn, *J.A.M.A.*, **112,** 7 (1939).
6. R. F. Ogilvie, *Quart. J. Med.*, **4,** 345 (1935).
7. S. Sailer, F. Sandhofer, and H. Braunsteiner, *Metabolism*, **15,** 135 (1966).
8. H. C. Walker, *Arch. Intern. Med.*, **93,** 951 (1954).
9. M. G. Wohl, and R. S. Goodhart, Eds., *Modern Nutrition in Health and Disease*, 2nd Ed., Lea & Febiger, Philadelphia, 1960.
10. J. Hirsch and E. Gallian, *J. Lipid Res.*, **9,** 110 (1968).
11. B. Wait and L. J. Robert, *J. Am. Diet. Assoc.*, **8,** 209 (1932).
12. E. S. Eppright, V. D. Sidwell, and P. P. Swanson. *J. Nutr.*, **54,** 371 (1954).
13. F. P. Heald, *New Engl. J. Med.*, **268,** 192, January 24; 243, January 31; 299, February 7; 361, February 14 (1963).
14. M. C. Hampton, R. L. Huenemann, L. R. Shapiro, and B. W. Mitchell. *J. Am. Diet. Assoc.*, **50,** 385 (1967).
15. M. A. Wharton, *J. Am. Diet. Assoc.*, **42,** 306 (1963).
16. H. Bruch, In *Adolescence: Psychosocial Perspectives*, G. Caplan and S. Leborici, Eds., Basic Books, New York, 1969.
17. H. Bruch, In *Eating Disorders*, Basic Books, New York, p. 134, 1973.

12

Nutrition in Adolescents with Inflammatory Bowel Disease

MURRAY DAVIDSON, M.D.

State University of New York, Stony Brook

Very few disturbances of gastrointestinal function or abnormalities of nutrition have been established to be associated regularly with any of the various forms of inflammatory bowel disease. Therefore, few special dietary maneuvers appear to be justified. Nevertheless many physicians plague their patients and interfere vigorously with diets. Patients are either urged to avoid certain "allergic" foods, spices, and roughage, because these are presumed to worsen the underlying disease process, or they are strongly encouraged to eat various rich but often unpalatable sources of protein and calories. The basis of most of these restrictions and supplements is questionable.

Too much dietary manipulation may be counterproductive in negativistic patients. We must be practical when dealing with children and adolescents. Good patient morale and appetite are often helpful allies in management of deficiencies, especially where poor intake may result not only from disease-induced anorexia but also from voluntary restrictions, either to avoid pain or as part of adolescent acting out. In general, we have always permitted most patients to eat whatever they desired to help maintain good intakes. A favorite aphorism we have long reiterated states that more protein is available from a hot dog that is ingested than from a steak left on one's plate. Although this policy has needed to be questioned on only very few occasions, it has proved helpful in the management of most patients.

This general attitude is altered in individual cases in whom certain types of troublesome symptomatology may respond to a dietary change. The most frequent alteration involves cow milk restriction.

Truelove and his associates demonstrated some years back, and have since steadfastly maintained, that antibody−antigen reactions to cow milk play a role in the genesis of inflammatory bowel disease (1, 2). A few patients with ulcerative colitis have hemagglutinating antibodies to tanned red cells coated with cow milk protein (3). However, these antibodies are present in normal persons; their titers in patients with ulcerative colitis do not correlate with the taking of milk or its withdrawal from the diet (4).

Although time has cast a good deal of doubt on the milk allergy thesis, certain considerations justify the continuation of a policy that the diet of virtually all newly encountered patients initially be unrestricted in all aspects except that it be free of cow milk and milk products. First, patients deserve the benefit of any doubt in the therapy of inflammatory bowel diseases and, even if somewhat weakened, the cow milk allergy argument has not been completely disproved. Second, other conditions associated with gastrointestinal losses of protein and blood have been attributed to the ingestion of cow milk protein (5−7). Third, one early aim of therapy is to avoid as many possible symptomatic pitfalls as possible. Withdrawal of lactose by prescription of the milk-free diet eliminates consideration of lactose intolerance in the symptomatology of the patient.

Our specific dietary advice at this juncture proscribes all forms of milk, butter, cream, cheese, and cooked or processed foods that contain any of milk, skim milk, whey, casein, or lactose. Patients are taught to avoid the hidden sources of milk, for example, when used as fillers in luncheon meats. Once the patient has been observed for a few months and the clinical picture is stabilized, milk products are gradually reintroduced and the effects are constantly evaluated. Whole milk is the last to be permitted. Most of the time it is tolerated well and no questions are raised about related symptoms. However, if there is increase in hematochezia or in diarrhea at any point during the reintroductions, careful clinical trials of withdrawals and feedings are carried out in an attempt to establish possible causal relationships. Very rarely a patient with ulcerative colitis is apparently able to tolerate milk products but experiences an increase in bleeding with whole milk. Such a patient may then continue through adolescence to take processed cheeses and foods cooked with milk as the sole sources of cow milk protein.

If, instead of bleeding, diarrhea or abdominal pain recur during milk reintroduction, appropriate serum tolerance or hydrogen breath tests are performed with a standardized lactose dose. We cannot be certain about whether the 10 to 15% of our patients who prove to be lactase deficient are so chiefly because of their ethnic propensities, since so many are of Ashkenazi Jewish extraction, or because of the influence of the disease. These patients are advised to limit their diets to soybean milk and to substitute foods such as soybean "ice cream." They are all treated with increased vitamin D and calcium supplements. We also teach them that symptoms derived from lactose ingestion, while troublesome, do not worsen the disease. Even the most intolerant individual retains the ability to digest some lactose. The larger the quantity ingested, the more that passes undigested to the colon for fermentation, the greater the resultant osmotic load, the more likely the individual is to have osmotic diarrhea or severe distension and abnormal discomfort. It is therefore reasonable for each individual with lactase insufficiency empirically to discover his or her own level of lactose intolerance and to balance symptomatology with desires. Most lactase deficient individuals are comfortably able to ingest limited quantities of foods made with milk. In social situations they display selectivity, merely tasting certain troublemakers, eating a bit more of others, occasionally splurging with the expectation of a loose stool, while almost always avoiding whole milk as a beverage.

For the large majority of inflammatory bowel disease patients who do not prove to be milk intolerant as it is reintroduced into their diets, we not only permit free intake but actually encourage those with poor weight gains to take extra milk as a caloric source. We usually prescribe as a basic daily allotment a quart of whole milk into which the skim milk powder equivalent to one quart has been suspended. Two 8-ounce glasses of the mixture are taken with meals. The other two are utilized for between meal or prebedtime supplements. One of these is whipped into a rich drink with a beaten whole egg, flavored syrup of the patient's choice, and malted milk powder. The second is mixed with a scoop of ice cream. This pattern of enriched milk supplements adds more than 1500 calories daily without imposing the prescription-type low-residue preparations which are often less acceptable. Nevertheless, we do not urge this dietary maneuver on any normally growing patient whose intake one must assume to be adequate.

Other dietary modifications that we employ are offered to very much more limited groups of patients and only on specific indications. In occasional patients with large bowel disease who are troubled with severe urgency or diarrhea, or among those with small bowel inflammation who experience annoying peristalic rushes, exclusion of such bowel stimulants as cold drinks, citrus juices, carbonated beverages, cocoa, and chocolate may be hlpful.

Patients with Crohn's disease of the small bowel may develop bile acid insufficiency by various mechanisms. Extensive disease of the distal ileum may preclude absorption of conjugated bile acids and may thus lead to an interruption of the normal enterohepatic circulation. Surgical resection of this area makes the defect permanent. Bile acid deficiency may also be associated with stasis from strictures and obstructions. Proximal excessive bacterial overgrowth or pileup of high concentrations of nonabsorbable antimicrobials leads to intraluminal deconjugation of bile acids and interferes with their normal absorption in the ileum. Whatever the underlying cause, the passage of unabsorbed bile acids to the colon will result in increase of cyclic AMP and leads to diarrhea by interfering with resorption of sodium and water. Binding of the bile acids by cholestyramine improves such diarrhea in some instances. However, many patients are unwilling to take the 8–12 g/day which is usually required and prefer to suffer the diarrhea. Patients with ileal resections of greater than 100 cm not only will usually not receive relief from cholestyramine binding of bile acids but it may frequently aggravate their steatorrhea. In these instances bacterial hydroxylation of certain of the unabsorbed fatty acids, for example, production of ricinoleic acid (castor oil), contributes to the diarrhea mechanism.

Calcium and magnesium losses are also increased in the face of the steatorrhea. These losses are aggravated by steroid administration. Signs of deficiency of these minerals may range from increased muscle weakness, irritability, positive Chvostek and Trousseau signs, and overt tetany to frank seizures.

Dietary measures to counteract bile acid losses, steatorrhea, and selective mineral losses include attempts to limit bile acid and fat losses by using medium chain triglycerides. However, these preparations are often poorly tolerated because of unacceptable tastes and because they may not help with diarrhea. Medium chain triglyceride preparations frequently contain considerable lactose and may induce symptoms in the presence of lactase deficiency. Prescription of a low fat diet with supplemental calcium and/or magnesium and increased vitamin D intake may be the preferable treatment.

Monthly injections of vitamin B_{12} may be called for with ileal insufficiency in severe disease. Resection of the distal ileum to cure such disease solves some problems but induces permanent vitamin B_{12} malabsorption, which requires lifelong continuation of the B_{12} injections. In instances of small intestinal obstruction, prescription of low residue intake means elimination of all fruits and vegetables to some physicians and may lead to low folic acid intake.

Iron deficiency may occur in malabsorption, as part of the acute blood loss in ulcerative colitis, with more chronic occult blood loss in any form of inflammatory bowel disease, and with the intestinal mucosal damage from cow milk. In all of these instances oral medicinal iron may be helpful. However, in the anemia associated with the chronic inflammatory picture of some patients with Crohn's disease, prescription of additional oral iron is of limited value. This pattern of anemia, although it is associated with low serum iron and low serum transferrin and other proteins, occurs in the face of adequate bone marrow iron stores.

Another mineral deficiency that is regularly associated with poor serum protein levels is that of zinc. This deficiency has been reported in patients with Crohn's disease and in certain other conditions associated with poor appetite and lack of growth (8). The question has been raised whether zinc deficiency is a cause of, or is a result of, poor intake, or of excessive losses in Crohn's disease. Despite the open question, the deficiency is not demonstrable except in a limited number of patients. In these instances medicinal zinc supplements are indicated.

Recently, a good deal of nutritional interest has been focused on the important problem of growth retardation. Many children and adolescents with inflammatory bowel disease exhibit retarded growth in height with delay in maturation of bone and secondary sexual characteristics (9, 10). The generalization that the degree of retardation usually correlates with the severity of clinical course and with the extent of bowel involvement often does not apply. The precise basis and mechanism of growth retardation remains uncertain and this serious problem is difficult to treat.

It is not uncommon to encounter growth failure preceding by years other clinical evidence of gastrointestinal disease. Of 130 patients with inflammatory bowel disease under 21 years of age, McCaffery et al. found 22 in whom growth failure was so severe that they were 2 standard deviations below the mean height for age (10). Nineteen of these patients had Crohn's disease; three had ulcerative colitis. A number of authors point out the greater likelihood of growth interference among patients with Crohn's disease than among those with ulcerative colitis (9, 11–13).

Increased incidence of the problem among patients with Crohn's disease suggests that defects in intestinal absorption may be at fault. Six of 11 patients studied by Beeken showed abnormal vitamin B_{12} absorption and low serum folate and iron levels; three patients had abnormal xylose absorption (14). Bacterial overgrowth in the upper small intestine has been found in 30% of such patients (15). Excessive losses of blood and protein in stools, and hypoalbuminemia are common (16).

However, in many other children and adolescents with growth failure and Crohn's disease, no defect in absorptive function is demonstrable.

Endocrine failure has therefore been suggested as a possible contributing factor to the poor growth. Findings such as reduced urinary gonadotropins and poor growth hormone release following insulin-induced hypoglycemia have been cited as etiologic factors (10). Nevertheless, such defects are probably nonspecific and are seen in children with maternal deprivation (17) or with protein-calorie malnutrition (18). Normal or elevated basal levels of growth hormone, exaggerated responses to sleep and to propranolol plus glucagon, and normal thyroid function are found in children with inflammatory bowel disease (19, 20); such results make a primary endocrine abnormality an unlikely cause of the growth failure, especially since exogenously administered growth hormone does not improve growth in such patients (21).

End organ resistance to the effects of growth hormone on the faulty release of somatomedin may be at fault. It is of interest that somatomedin levels have been found to be depressed in some malnourished children (22). Indeed, it may be that the growth abnormalities found in Crohn's disease reflect significant malnutrition. Large doses of corticosteroids such as are often used to control inflammatory bowel disease may also contribute to growth failure. Increased excretion of nitrogen occurs after administration of pharmacological doses of corticosteroids (23). Nevertheless, one group that has reported growth retardation in adolescents with inflammatory bowel disease also maintains that patients may be induced to grow despite high-dose steroid therapy, presumably because of the suppression of inflammatory activity (24). The controlling factor for growth in such patients may actually be increased caloric intake, but this has not been adequately studied.

Data on the effects of surgery on growth are conflicting. For reasons that are still unclear, growth after surgery in childhood and adolescence sometimes remains depressed in patients with Crohn's disease, although successes have been achieved, particularly in young patients operated on before puberty (25). The response to surgery (total proctocolectomy with ileostomy) is usually dramatic among patients with severe growth failure in ulcerative colitis, especially when surgery is performed prior to the onset of puberty (26).

Most reports and reviews recently have emphasized that nutritional deficiency is the significant factor in the failure of growth and maturation in children with inflammatory bowel disease. Neither endocrine dysfunction nor malabsorption appears to account for the severe growth failure (27–29). A variety of mechanisms, including continuing losses from inflamed bowel mucosa, bacterial overgrowth in obstructed loops with subsequent steatorrhea, fistulous short circuits, anorexia, and poor intake to avoid pain, appear to lead to the chronic malnutrition. The most desirable way to provide nutrition to the sick child is by means of a palatable, balanced, and nutritious diet. This obvious point bears reemphasis because of the attitudes of children, particularly adolescents, toward food. Special diets designed to provide increased protein or specific fat sources may be unpalatable and have the potential in some patients to suppress appetite.

Low residue diets have been administered as the only food intake in ulcerative colitis as well as in Crohn's disease. The treatment was initially introduced to reduce bowel activity and hopefully to reduce inflammation. Some patients demonstrated that they not only felt better but were able as a result of the reduced bulk and improved nutrition offered over a period of months to close fistulae if they existed, and/or to experience marked gain in weight and height.

The use of total parenteral nutrition either via a central catheter or via peripheral vein with calories supplied in large amounts for a month or more has been reported as improving the nutritional status in debilitated patients with inflammatory bowel disease (30, 31). The goal of parenteral nutritional therapy is avoidance or reversal of protein-calorie malnutrition and restoration of body cell mass in preparation for surgery. However, in some of these patients growth arrest was subsequently reported to be reversed following this treatment. It was suggested that growth retardation might be a major indication for primary parenteral nutritional therapy.

Effective utilization of protein depends upon the availability of fuel substrates to meet the caloric requirements for its synthesis. If not enough calories in the form of endogenous lipid and/or carbohydrates are provided, amino acids will be oxidized for energy and negative nitrogen balance results. Negative nitrogen balance exists during periods of stress as protein is catabolized from the body cell mass. Positive nitrogen balance is achieved when urinary nitrogen is equivalent to or less than the nitrogen administered orally or parenterally. Maintenance of positive nitrogen balance requires an appropriate ratio of grams of nitrogen to calories, in the ranges of 1:100 to 1:200. Therefore, 1 g of nitrogen (equivalent to 6.25 g of protein) requires from 100 to 200 calories of nonprotein to reduce significant nitrogen loss.

Protein/carbohydrate infusions in patients on prolonged parenteral nutrition may be supplemented by intravenous lipid emulsions to prevent essential fatty acid deficiency. Lipids may also serve as an alternative source of nonprotein calories. The commercially available solutions, Intralipid 10% IV Fat Emulsion® or 10% Liposyn®, consist of soybean or safflower oil in an egg yolk phospholipid emulsifier and provide 1.1 cal/cc. The daily dosage should not exceed 2.5 g/kg in 24 h in adults and 4 g/kg in 24 h in children. It should make up no more than 60% of the total caloric input.

REFERENCES

1. K. B. Taylor and S. C. Truelove, *Br. Med. J.*, **2**, 924 (1961).
2. R. Wright and S. C. Truelove, *Br. Med. J.*, **2**, 138 (1965).
3. R. Wright and S. C. Truelove, *Br. Med. J.*, **2**, 142 (1965).
4. S. C. Kraft and J. Kirsner, *Gastroenterology*, **60**, 922 (1971).
5. J. D. Gryboski, F. Burkle, and R. Hillman, *Pediatrics*, **38**, 29 (1966).
6. T. A. Waldmann, R. D. Wochner, L. Laster, et al., *New Engl. J. Med.*, **276**, 761 (1967).
7. P. Kuitunen, J. K. Visakorpi, E. Savilahti, et al., *Arch. Dis. Child*, **50**, 351 (1975).
8. N. W. Solomons and R. L. Rosenfield, *Pediat. Res.*, **10**, 923 (1976).
9. E. H. Sobel, F. N. Silverman, and C. M. Lee, Jr., *Am. J. Dis. Child.*, **103**, 569 (1962).
10. T. D. McCaffery, K. Naskr, A. M. Lawrence, et al., *Pediatrics*, **45**, 386 (1970).
11. M. Berger, D. Gribetz, and B. I. Korelitz, *Pediatrics*, **55**, 459 (1965).
12. M. Davidson, A A. Bloom, and M. M. Kugler, *Pediatrics*, **67**, 471 (1965).
13. B. Cavell, H. Hildebrand, G. G. Meeuwisse, and B. Lindquist, *Clin. Gastroent.*, **6**, 481 (1977).
14. W. L. Beeken, *Pediatrics*, **52**, 69 (1973).
15. W. L. Beeken and R. E. Kanich, *Gastroenterology*, **65**, 390 (1973).
16. W. L. Beeken, H. J. Busch, and D. L. Sylvester, *Gastroenterology*, **62**, 207 (1972).
17. G. F. Powell, J. A. Brasel, and R. M. Blizzard, *New Engl. J. Med.*, **276**, 1271 (1967).
18. D. J. Becker, B. L. Pimstone, and J. D. Hansen, *Pediat. Res.*, **9**, 35 (1975).
19. R. W. Gotlin and R. S. Dubos, *Gut*, **14**, 191 (1973).
20. A. Tenore, J. S. Parks, R. T. Kirkland, et al., *Pediat. Res.*, **9**, 309 (1975).
21. T. D. McCaffery, K. Nasr, A. M. Lawrence, et al., *Am. J. Dig. Dis.*, **19**, 411 (1974).
22. D. B. Grant, J. Hambley, and D. Becker, et al., *Arch. Dis. Child.*, **48**, 596 (1973).
23. R. W. Wannemacher, Jr., "Protein Metabolism," in H. Ghadimi, Ed., *Total Parenteral Nutrition*, Wiley, New York, 1975, p. 85.
24a. E. J. Burbige, S. S. Huange, and T. M. Bayless, *Pediatrics*, **55**, 866 (1975).
24b. T. M. Bayless, personal communication.
25. C. F. Frey and D. K. Weaver, *Arch. Surg.*, **104**, 416 (1972).
26. M. Berger, D. Gribetz, and B. I. Korelitz, *Pediatrics*, **55**, 459 (1975).
27. M. I. Cohen, S. J. Boley, P. R. Winslow, and F. Daum, *Pediatric Res.*, **7**, 336 (1973).
28. T. Layden, J. Rosenberg, B. Nemchausky, C. Elson, and I. H. Rosenberg, *Gastroenterology*, **70**, 107 (1976).
29. D. G. Kelts, R. J. Grand, G. Shen, J. B. Watkins, S. L. Werlin, and C. Boehme, *Gastroenterology*, **76**, 720 (1979).
30. R. H. Driscoll and I. H. Rosenberg, *Med. Clin. N. Am.*, **62**, 185 (1978).
31. C. T. Strobel, W. J. Byrne, and M. E. Ament, *Gastroenterology*, **77**, 272 (1979).

13

New Concepts in Atherosclerosis as it Applies to Adolescents

FELIX P. HEALD, M.D.

University of Maryland, School of Medicine, Baltimore, Maryland

For the last 30 years ischemic heart disease has been determined to be the largest cause of death in the United States. Of the 1.9 billion deaths in 1976, nearly one-third were attributed to ischemic heart disease. Various terms such as arteriosclerotic, coronary artery, and ischemic heart disease have been used to denote the clinical manifestations of atherosclerosis. Since 1969, the preferred term has been ischemic heart disease. Basically, this is a process in which the lumen of the artery becomes increasingly narrow from the accumulation of smooth muscle cells, connective tissue matrix, and lipids. As a result, arterial circulation is diminished, resulting in ischemic disease of the brain, legs, and heart. Although this process is not fully understood, it does involve the growth of a focal tumor of cells called an athroma in the arterial wall. In its earliest stages, the process consists of smooth muscle cells, cholesterol, and cellular debris. Later its structure is complicated by growth of fiberous tissue and subsequently by deposits of calcium. This process may begin early in life, even in infancy, and progresses slowly over decades. Distressingly it has been noted with increasing frequency in young adult life, although clinical disease is evident primarily in middle and late adult life. Why should we be discussing this particular disorder in a conference on nutrition of adolescents?

Unfortunately, this process has been noted consistently in children to a limited degree, but during adolescence there is a very rapid rise in the amount of fatty streaking, particularly in the aorta.

PREVALENCE IN CHILDREN

Holman in 1958 using autopsy specimens from New Orleans, reported the rather startling observation that there was considerable acceleration of fatty streaking during adolescence (1). Although there is some evidence of fatty streaking, even in infancy, its most dramatic increase occurred during adolescence. Subsequently, Strong (2), who was associated with Dr. Holman in the original research, repeated the original study. The observations began in 1960 and lasted until 1968. Two thousand seven hundred persons were studied in a similar manner as reported in 1958 during which time they again noted the rather striking black–white difference, black males in the 10–14 age group having three times as much fatty streaking as white males. At the same age, a similar difference was noted among white versus black females. From 15 to 24 years the white male had almost caught up with his black counterpart in the amount of fatty streaking found in the aorta. Therefore, there is substantial evidence that the origin of atherosclerosis may be deeply rooted in the second decade of life.

THEORIES OF ATHEROSCLEROSIS

There are basically three major theories concerning the etiology and explanation of the process of arteriosclerosis.

Monoclonal Theory

This recent hypothesis, proposed by Benditt and Benditt (3), supposes that each lesion of atherosclerosis is derived from a single smooth muscle cell which serves as a parent for the remaining proliferating cells. The Benditts took advantage of the observation that arteriosclerotic plaques frequently appeared as masses surrounded by large areas of normal tissue. Using the biochemical techniques of measuring glucose-6-phosphate dehydrase isomer, the Benditts identified the clonal cellular state of the atherosclerotic lesion. In humans, the cellular proliferation appears to be monoclonal. This observation will be of great help in identifying animal models that are cellularly analogous to the human model. The Benditts' observations are the basis for the "cancer theory of atherogenesis."

Clonal-Senescence Theory

This theory (4) has its roots in aging, which is a well recognized risk factor in atherosclerosis. Human cells have a limited ability to replicate which varies inversely with age. This age-related decline in ability to reproduce is greater for cells in the abdominal aorta than for those in the thoracic aorta. Of more than passing interest is the fact that atherosclerosis is more common in the abdominal aorta than in the thoracic aorta. On the basis of these observations, Martin and Sprague proposed that the declining is linked to the development of atherogenesis.

The Response to Injury Theory

The response to injury hypothesis dates back to 1857, more than 130 years ago (Virchow), and recently has been reviewed by Ross and Glomset (5). Over the years this theory has been modified and expanded by a number of investigators. The basis for the hypothesis lies in the similarity between atherosclerosis and the response of arteries to experimental mechanical injury. Factors such as hyperlipidemia, hormone dysfunction, increased turbulence resulting from hypertension, and angiotoxic factors may injure the endothelium and alter the nature of this barrier to the contents of plasma. These factors alter the endothelial cells or endothelial cell–connective tissue relationships, permitting detachment of endothelial cells from the arterial wall. This focal desquamation of the endothelium exposes the underlying connective tissue to platelets and other elements in plasma. Subsequently platelets adhere to the subendothelium collagen; infiltration of the injured site with lipoproteins and other plasma constituents, such as hormones, begins at the site of injury. Focal proliferation of the arterial smooth muscle cells results in the formation of large amounts of connective tissue matrix by these cells. The final step in this process is a deposition of lipids both within the cells and in the surrounding connective tissue matrix. With healing, the endothelial barrier gets reestablished and the lesions regress provided the angiotoxic event is limited. This sequence of events may repeat itself, with further injury resulting in further proliferation of smooth muscle cells and accumulation of connective tissue. Lipid deposition may occur if the injury is continuous and/or repeated and particularly if a state of hypercholesterolemia exists. Thus, there is a critical balance between angiotoxic injury and repair. Any disturbance in this critical balance determines whether the lesions enlarge, remain constant, or regress. It is this reaction to injury that characterizes the fatty streak found primarily in the aorta, the prime lesion noted during the juvenile period.

CHOLESTEROL

There may be a number of ways in which chronic hyperlipidemia and/or hypercholesterolemia may injure the endothelium. It is not clear whether the injury results from a sustained increase in the cholesterol pool or from more complicated effects of chronic hyperlipidemia or altered lipoproteins upon the endothelial cells. It is appropriate to recall the work of Ross and Parker, who observed that the effect of a single mechanical injury to aortic endothelium in the absence of hyperlipidemia resulted in smooth muscle proliferation identical to the preatherosclerotic fiber muscular lesion seen in man (6). This lesion reaches its maximum size 3 months after injury and largely disappears in 6 months. In those experimental animals rendered chronically hyperlipidemic for 6 months after the mechanical deendothelialization, the lesions instead of regressing either remained unchanged or in some instances increased in size. As one would predict, large amorphous intercellular lipid deposits were present and lipid accumulated as amorphous droplets in the surrounding tissue. These and other observations suggest that chronic hyperlipidemia prevents lesion regression and augments lipid deposition, hence promotes atherosclerotic progression.

If hyperlipidemia is a facilitator in the development of atherosclerosis, what is the relationship between dietary cholesterol, total serum cholesterol, and atherosclerosis. Epidemiological studies of human populations focusing on total serum cholesterol have shown a powerful relationship between this lipid and the development of coronary disease. If this link could be established, then the dietary role of cholesterol and a logical course for prevention would be established.

CHOLESTEROL AND ATHEROSCLEROSIS

Cholesterol, particularly cholesterol esters, are the principal lipid compound in atherosclerotic lesions. Epidemiological studies have repeatedly demonstrated the association of elevated total serum cholesterol with coronary artery disease. Kannel (7) has pointed out that the risk is not confined to those with hypercholesterolemia, but is stratified within the population, with the risk rising with cholesterol values varying from the lowest to the highest. However, cholesterol risk must be taken in context with other risk factors. As age increases the influence of cholesterol as a predictor of coronary disease weakens. Other strong risk factors identified in the Framingham study were glucose intolerance, hypertension, cigarette smoking, and left ventricular hypertrophy (7). This study strongly demonstrates that the risk varies at any level of serum cholesterol according to the dose of other risk factors. Thus, cholesterol, though important, is not the absolute determinant of clinical heart disease. Evidence particularly from the Framingham study indicates that the bulk of coronary disease in the current epidemic is found among those individuals in the mid portion of the bell-shaped curve for serum cholesterol levels. There is essentially no difference in serum cholesterol in middle-aged men between those who are going to have clinical coronary disease and those who are not. Total serum cholesterol, then, is not an absolute predictor of clinical disease. Either one of two things is true. There may be fractions of cholesterol in the lipoproteins which are more predictive than total serum cholesterol. This may be the case, particularly with LDL and HDL. These lipoprotein fractions show the greatest promise of all the protein carriers of cholesterol in having some predictive value for clinical coronary artery disease. That is, those individuals with lower amounts of cholesterol LDL or greater amounts of HDL cholesterol appear to have less clinical atherosclerotic disease.

Most of the cholesterol in the blood is carried in the low density lipoprotein (LDL), and has a high correlation with total serum cholesterol. A large amount of cholesterol in LDL fraction is a powerful predictor of risk for arterial disease in subjects less than 50 years of age. Thus, cholesterol plays an important, though not an all inclusive, role in the development of arterial disease in humans. Over the age of 50, total serum cholesterol has little, if any, association with clinical events. A combination of elevated LDL and a low HDL appears to be associated with clinical disease from age 50 on.

High density lipoprotein carries about 25% of total serum cholesterol. It appears that HDL is a major carrier of cholesterol from cells to the liver for further metabolism and elimination from the body by biliary metabolism. There is data to suggest an inverse relationship between the level of HDL and total body cholesterol. Further, the levels of HDL in blood appear to correlate with clinical disease. High levels appear to be "protective" whereas low levels are correlated with atherosclerotic artery disease (7). Or the other possibility is that there is some chemical (trans fatty acids) in the diet which interferes with cholesterol metabolism, as has been proposed by Mann, in such a way that the total body pool of cholesterol is increased (8). He proposed that some oxides of cholesterol or trans fatty acids impair the activity of 7-alpha-hydroxylase, the rate limiting enzyme in cholesterol catabolism. This inhibition could lead to a larger body pool of cholesterol and hence to hypercholesterolemia.

DIETARY CHOLESTEROL AND BLOOD CHOLESTEROL

Unfortunately, this relationship has not been proven. In fact, the opposite is true. In two large studies, the Framingham (9) study and the Tecumseh (10) study, levels of serum lipids were found to be unrelated to dietary practice. In fact during this century (1909) the dietary level of cholesterol intake has remained steady at 600 mg/day. During this time when cholesterol levels in the United States remained steady, a sharp rise in coronary artery disease has developed which peaked in the 1960s. Even more interesting, since the mid 1960s there has been a clearcut decrease in clinical coronary disease in this country. This decrease has no real explanation, although unlikely related to dietary cholesterol currently identified as a risk factor in the diet. Further evidence on the role of dietary cholesterol in arteriosclerosis comes from clinical trials of two kinds. The first type of study consisted of subjects who were initially free of coronary disease (Framingham). The second group were those subjects known to have coronary disease in whom dietary practices of intervention were introduced. Basically, as a result no dietary treatment has been shown to be effective for the prevention or treatment of coronary disease (12–14). It is known that drugs such as cholestramine, cholefibrate, and niacin could reduce cholesteremia by 15 to 20%. Yet in clinical trials so far neither has had a measurable effect on the appearance of coronary heart disease after 5 years of intervention and observation. This evidence is important since drug therapy is about twice as effective as dietary therapy in lowering serum cholesterol levels (15, 16).

Summarizing our discussion so far, some atherosclerosis is found in all human societies examined. The technologically advanced societies have a higher cholesterolemia and their atherosclerosis is more xanthomatous and more obstructive. However, within such societies, individual total blood cholesterol values are not accurate predictors of coronary disease, although cholesterol lipoprotein carriers offer better association with clinical disease. And, feeding studies indicate that the elevation may not be due to higher dietary intake. Another possibility is that there is something noxious in the diet that is more angiotoxic than pure cholesterol itself. It is this latter concept that I would like to explore with you in the last part of our discussion.

ANGIOTOXICITY IN JUVENILE DIETS

As our earlier discussion indicated there were two reasons to suspect that factors other than cholesterol itself is the major cause of the current epidemic of atherosclerosis and lead to the search for angiotoxic chemicals. First is the typical reaction to injury that is so characteristic of human atherosclerosis, suggesting some noxious agent had injured the aorta cells. Second is the lack of strong evidence that dietary cholesterol per se was the most important risk factor. One needs to turn to the earlier history of research in atherosclerosis, to the original experiment when Anitschkow in 1913 fed cholesterol dissolved in vegetable oil to rabbits (17, 18). These animals developed atherosclerotic lesions now considered to be typical of this disorder. This experiment was the beginning of a long series of animal studies involving cholesterol feeding which resulted in hypercholesterolemia, the basis of our current concept of atherosclerosis. As early as 1904 sterol chemists had shown the labile nature of cholesterol; that is, it is oxidized readily. In the 1950s Swenk attempted to feed some of the oxidation products of cholesterol to produce atherosclerosis (19). This was not successful, which may have been the result of an inappropriate dose or an improper choice of the cholesterol derivative from among the many oxidation products then well known to sterol chemists. Van Lier and Smith (20) in the late 1960s had identified 12 of 32 known oxidation products of cholesterol in the aortas of older adults at autopsy. Imai and Taylor reported their studies, which strongly suggest that the oxidation products of cholesterol may play a significant role in the pathogenesis of the current epidemic of atherosclerosis (21, 22). In the first place even newly purchased chemical cholesterol contains about 5% oxidation products and after five years 40% of the cholesterol sitting on the shelf has been converted to oxidation products. The most prevalent is 25-hydroxy-cholesterol, and it by chance is the most cytotoxic of the oxidation products. Imai's initial cytotoxicity studies were on whole animals, which included the pig and rabbit. Their subsequent tissue culture studies of smooth muscle cells can be summarized as follows. They took USP cholesterol and purified it. The investigators then fed both the residue from purification and the purified cholesterol to animals in an acute toxicity experiment. The residue produced an increased frequency of dead aortic smooth muscle cells, including focal edema, in the rabbit 24 hours after gavage. Purified cholesterol fed in similar amounts did not increase the number of dead whole cells. When the concentrate was fed to the animals over a prolonged period of time (a total dose of 2 g/kg over 7 weeks) the animals developed diffuse fibromuscular scars without foam cells or hypercholesterolemia. Purified cholesterol at the same dosage level produced no demonstrable effect. The investigators were able to iden- tify from their USP chemical cholesterol by appropriate separation techniques eight oxidation products, which again were in agreement with those identified by Smith both in chemical cholesterol and in human aortas. Taylor, utilizing the model of cultured aortic smooth muscle cells, showed that 25-hydroxy-cholesterol was the most potent cytotoxic agent—far more toxic than pure cholesterol. Other spontane- ously occurring contaminates of cholesterol were cholestane 3-beta, 5-alpha, and 6-beta-triol seemed to be the next most toxic (23). The literature suggests that endogenously produced cholesterol is protected from auto-oxidation in the body by antioxidants. Our own research group visited the Albany laboratories in 1973 and were aware of their early work in oxidation products. Since then, we have begun to look at oxidation products in the aortas of adolescents and adults and have confirmed the work of Smith, finding the similar pattern of oxidation products in the aortas of adults, the primary one being 25-hydroxy- cholesterol, the oxide most cytotoxic. These oxidation products are located in the fatty streaks and are absent in the normal portion of the aorta. We recently completed work on looking at oxidation products in the fatty streaks of the aortas of teenagers. To be sure they are found in the same pattern as adults—the most prevalent one being 25-hydroxy- cholesterol. Thus, it appears that the fatty streaks of teenagers have a similar pattern of deposition of oxidation products of cholesterol as adults. This then raises the question whether the oxidation products of cholesterol are the cytotoxic element which initiates the arterial injury?

What implications does this rather unexpected set of findings have for our current concepts of atherosclerosis? First, it may mean that all of the feeding experiments to date which utilize USP grade cholesterol stored in air-room temperature will have to be reevaluated. In the majority of instances the experimental diet probably contained significant quantities of oxidized sterols, which have a striking lethal effect on aortic intimal cells. This is combined with the fact that cholesterol, either endogeously synthesized or chemically isolated pure cholesterol, is not strongly cytotoxic. However, the combination of pure cholesterol and its toxic derivatives may be highly atherogenic.

What implication does this have for human disease? The missing link of course is where do these products come from? For example, powdered eggs have significant amounts of oxidation products of cholesterol. Such studies have been in the literature since the 1960s and our own laboratory oxidation products of cholesterol have been identified in our own experimental powdered egg diet. Forty percent of the eggs in this country are consumed as powdered egg. The processing of powdered eggs makes it highly likely that oxidation products will result in the commercial product. Taylor's group has also isolated derivatives of cholesterol oxidation products from two readily available retail packaged foods that contained dried whole egg or egg yolks (22). One was a powdered custard mix and the other was a pancake mix. Another source of oxidized cholesterol is powdered whole milk, and even powdered nonfat milk may contain 10 mg of cholesterol per reconstituted quart. Smoked meat and smoked fish products may contain appreciable amounts of oxidation products. Cheese that is exposed to warm air for long periods of time during processing and later stored at room temperature may also contain significant quanitities of toxic cholesterol derivatives. Thus, the whole processing of cholesterol-containing foods in our diet may need to be clearly reevaluated in order to eliminate the amount of toxic oxidation products of cholesterol, such as 25-hydroxy-cholesterol. The proper preparation of food in the kitchen may also be an issue. Heat in the presence of oxygen can induce oxidation. Fresh eggs, as measured in our laboratory and by others, do not have oxidation products. Relevant to this discussion is the work of Pollak in 1958 (24). He demonstrated that different methods of egg preparation resulted in different cholesterol levels when the products of preparation were fed to rabbits. Fried or hard boiled eggs produced the highest cholesterol diets (10−14 times higher than normal), while scrambled or baked eggs increased 6−7 times, while soft boiled or raw eggs increased 3−4 times. Thus, food preparation in the kitchen may change the chemical nature of cholesterol and play a significant role in atherogenesis.

Finally, and briefly, a second potential factor in the juvenile atherosclerosis is that of vitamin D. Vanderveer in 1931 published the first paper linking hypervitaminosis D and arteriosclerosis (25). Recently, Kummerow has raised the specter of large amounts of vitamin D in the diets of humans coming from supplements in food and from animal sources. He has clearly demonstrated that experimental animals fed high doses of vitamin D will produce a diffuse fibrolastic intimal thickening not unlike that seen in plaques of thoracic aortas obtained as a byproduct of elective coronary bypass surgery. Vitamin D content of human tissue is somewhat higher than normally found in swine fed vitamin D at a level 14 times that normally recommended. Currently it is established that the vitamin D intake in pregnancy from all supplemented sources may average 2435 international units, which is about six times the National Research Council requirement. It has been estimated that the intake of vitamin D in infants is three times higher than that of adults. Thus, we are forced to speculate on the potential of vitamin D injury to the arterial intima during fetal life and infancy as another cytotoxic agent that children may be exposed to in their everyday lives. In summary,

1. The reaction to injury theory seems to fit the experimental data accurately as an explanation for the fatty streak atheroma formation.
2. Fatty streaking develops rapidly during adolescence.
3. Atheromatous clinical disease is characteristic of technologically advanced countries.
4. The dietary cholesterol theory explanation of this epidemic is not completely satisfactory.
5. Angiotoxic factors, particularly oxidative products of cholesterol, if confirmed by further investigation, may provide a reasonable explanation for arterial disease.
6. If this is true, technological refinements in processing cholesterol-containing foods are both indicated and realistic.

REFERENCES

1. R. L. Holman, H. C. McGill, J. P. Strong, and J. C. Geer, *Am. J. Pathol.*, **34,** 209 (1958).
2. J. P. Strong, C. Restrepo, and M. Guzman, *Lab. Invest.*, **39,** 364 (1978).

3. E. P. Benditt and J. M. Benditt, *Proc. Natl. Acad. Sci.*, **70**, 1753 (1973).

4. G. Martin, C. Ogburn, and C. Sprague, "Senescence and Vascular Disease," in V. J. Cristafalo, J. Roberts, and R. C. Adelman, Eds., *Exploration in Aging*, New York, Plenum, 1975, pp. 163–193.

5. R. Ross and J. A. Glomset, *New Engl. J. Med.*, **295**, 420 (1976).

6. R. Ross and L. Harker, *Science*, **193**, 1094 (1976).

7. W. B. Kannel, W. P. Catellli, and T. Gordon, *Ann. Int. Med.*, **90**, 85 (1979).

8. G. V. Mann, *New Engl. J. Med.*, **297**, 644 (1977).

9. W. B. Kannel and T. Gordon, The Framingham Diet Study: Diet and the Regulation of Serum Cholesterol (Sect. 24). Washington, D.C., Department of Health, Education and Welfare, 1970.

10. A. B. Nichols, C. Ravenscroft, D. E. Lamphiear, et al., *Am. J. Clin. Nutr.*, **29**, 1384 (1976).

11. F. A. Kummerow, *Am. J. Clin. Nutr.*, **32**, 58 (1979).

12. P. Leren, *Acta. Med. Scand.* (Suppl), **466**, 5 (1966).

13. S. Dayton and M. L. Pearce, *Am. J. Med.*, **46**, 751 (1964).

14. M. Miettinen, O. Turpeinen, M. J. Karvonen, et al., *Lancet*, **2**, 835 (1972).

15. Coronary Drug Project Research Group, *J.A.M.A.*, **231**, 360 (1975).

16. K. M. Detre and L. Shaw, *Circulation*, **50**, 998 (1974).

17. N. Anitschkow, *Ber. Ges. Russ. Arzte. Petersburg*, **80**, 1 (1912).

18. N. Anitschkow, *Beitr. Pathol. Anat. Allerg. Pathol.*, **56**, 379 (1913).

19. E. Schwenk, D. F. Stevens, and R. Altschul, *Proc. Soc. Exp. Biol. Med.*, **102**, 42 (1959).

20. L. L. Smith and J. E. Van Lier, *Atherosclerosis*, **12**, 1 (1970).

21. H. Imai, N. T. Werthessen, et al., *Science*, **207**, 651 (1980).

22. C. B. Taylor, S. K. Peng, N. T. Werthessen, et al., *Am. J. Clin. Nutr.*, **32**, 40 (1979).

23. S. K. Peng, C. B. Taylor, P. Tham, et al., *Arch. Pathol. Lab. Med.*, **102**, 57 (1978).

24. O. J. Pollak, *J. Am. Ger. Soc.*, **6**, 614 (1958).

25. H. L. Vanderveer, *Arch. Path.*, **12**, 941 (1931).

Index